The Fasting-Cure

E. H. Dewey

NOTES AND PRESS COMMENTS ON VOLUNTARY FASTS.

The first voluntary protracted fast for the cure of chronic ailing to reach the public prints as a matter of interesting news occurred in the case of Mr. C. C. H. Cowan, of Warrensburg, Ill., early in 1899. He had been on the two-meal plan for a time, and wishing for something more radical wrote to me as to his entering upon a fast. I probably wrote him as I now find it necessary to write all who feel that fasts are necessary and cannot have my personal care, "Go on a fast and stick to it until hunger comes or until your friends begin to suffer the pangs of sympathetic starvation; then compromise with the sin of ignorance by eating the least that will bring peace to their troubled souls."

The results were summed up by the *Morning-Herald Dispatch,* Decatur, Ill., April 16, 1899:

"A few years ago Dr. Tanner, in New York City, fasted for forty days and forty nights, and all the world wondered. Up to that time the feat was considered impossible. From day to day the papers told of his actions and his condition, and the entire people became deeply interested in the performance. Medical men and scientists became interested in the performance, and the laity watched the faster through curiosity. Tanner's accomplishment was considered marvellous by the medical profession and laymen alike, but Dr. Tanner has long since been a back number, and his performance is not now regarded as remarkable, although there are not many persons who would care to attempt the fast. Tanner was simply trying to prove that the thing could be done. He did it, and within a year the man who held the attention of the people of the country for forty days was a visitor to this city. What Tanner did has been more than accomplished by a Macon County man, but he went about his undertaking quietly, and the fact that he was fasting was known to only a few of his friends. The man is C.

C. H. Cowan, of Warrensburg, and for forty-two days and nights he abstained from the use of food in solid or liquid form. He began his fast on March 2 and broke it on the evening of April 13 at supper-time. With the exception of the loss of thirty pounds of flesh, which materially changed his personal appearance, Mr. Cowan shows no ill-effects of his undertaking. When he began he weighed one hundred and sixty-five pounds, and when he quit he weighed one hundred and thirty-five pounds. Before his fast he was inclined to be fleshy, and now, while still in fairly good flesh, his clothing manifests a desire not to hold close communion with his body. Mr. Cowan was in the city Saturday, and some of his friends did not know him. He related his experience to some of them, but he did this cautiously, and with the oft-expressed hope that the papers would not devote any attention to the affair, because he was not seeking and did not want notoriety. At different times during his fast the *Herald-Dispatch* has referred to the fact in short items. Cowan is a disciple of a Dr. Dewey, living at Meadville, Pa., who is an advocate of fasting as a means of curing many of the ills to which the body is heir. Dr. Dewey has many pamphlets touching the subject, and has also written some books for his belief, and his reasons have been made so plausible that a number of persons have coincided with him. Cowan says the efficacy of the treatment has been established in many instances, a fact that he can prove by ample testimony. During his long abstinence from food he had numerous letters and telegrams from Dr. Dewey, encouraging him in the undertaking. When asked why he had fasted, Cowan explained that for years he had suffered from chronic nasal and throat catarrh which would not yield to medical treatment. His appetite was splendid, and he ate many things that he really did not want. He read Dr. Dewey's ideas, and became convinced that his system needed general overhauling, and that this could be accomplished through faithful adherence to the theory of Dr. Dewey. One of these theories is to the effect that fasting rests the brain, which is ofttimes overworked as a result of heavy feeding. It is also supposed that the body throws off old mucous membrane of the stomach and bowels, and that these are immediately supplanted by new lining. Believing that he could get rid of his catarrhal trouble and get the new lining referred to, Cowan decided to fast, and without noise about the matter he commenced, and up to Thursday evening he did not allow a bite of food to pass his lips. The only thing that he took was water. Of this he did not drink much, and he claims that he suffered no pain or pangs of hunger. Looking at the matter now, it does not seem to have been much of an accomplishment. After he once got started he said it was an easy matter to carry out his plan except for the worry of his family and some of his friends. They thought that he was losing his mind and tried to induce him to relinquish his idea, but he took some of them under his wing and reasoned with them on the beauties of the treatment, expounded the strong points, gave them reasons, showed them testimony of others, and kept on fasting. When he began he had no idea that he would continue for forty days; but as he progressed he had no desire for food, and therefore did not desist. Thursday evening he began to feel hungry, and that night he ate a reasonably good supper. The return of hunger, according to his theories, was the signal of the return of health. He feels confident that his stomach has been relined, and for the present he knows that his catarrh has left him. He is a firm believer in the new method of curing bodily ailments, and says that during his fast he was able to be around the village of Warrensburg every day, and was able to perform his duties. His abstinence from food apparently has not weakened his constitution. Since breaking his fast he has partaken sparingly of food. Cowan's friends are very much interested in the recital of his experience."

It so chanced that during this fast much more than his ordinary business came to him, and without the least inability to perform it. I saw him several months later, and found his physical condition seemingly perfect. He had found out that for the best working conditions a nap at noon was better than even a light luncheon, and that one meal a day taken after his business was over was the best practice. This fast was not in the right locality to excite the attention it deserved.

The second voluntary fast was destined to reach the ends of the earth through the public prints. The following appeared in the *New York Press* of June 6, 1899:

"Twenty-eight days without nourishment and without letting up for a moment on the daily routine of his business is the unequalled record of Milton Rathbun, a hay and grain dealer at No. 453 Fourth Avenue, and living in Mount Vernon. He is a man of wealth, has many employés, and has been in the same business in this city for thirty-nine years.

"He fasted because he wanted to reduce his weight, fearing that its gradual increase might bring on apoplexy. He succeeded in his efforts. He weighed two hundred and ten pounds when he stopped eating; when he resumed he tipped the scales at one hundred and sixty-eight pounds, a loss of forty-two pounds of flesh.

"Mr. Rathbun's description of how he felt as the days and weeks wore along and the pounds of avoirdupois slipped away one by one is interesting. The remarkable point about it is that he continued his work and kept well. He gave his account of it yesterday to a reporter for *The Press*. Mr. Rathbun is known by the business men for blocks around his own place of business, and they all know of his fast.

"Every day his friends would come in and talk to him about it. At first they told him he was foolish; that nobody could fast that length of time, much less continue his work without interruption. Then as the days went on and he kept up without a break they began to be frightened.

"A crowd would gather about him every night at 6.30 o'clock, when he would leave his office, for that was his hour for weighing. Some days he would lose two or three pounds from the weight of the day before; some days only one, but always something. And as the record was scored up on the book each night his friends would shake their heads and warn him to beware.

"Finally, on the fifteenth day, his friends and employés got together and made up their minds that something had to be done. They were afraid that Rathbun would die. They appointed a committee to wait on him in his office and beg him to eat something. The committee took dainties to Mr. Rathbun, told him their fears, and offered the good things to tempt him, but all to no purpose.

"It was the night of April 23 that Mr. Rathbun took his last bit of nourishment. He made no attempt to eat a large meal in preparation for his fast. He ate his regular supply just as if he had meant to continue eating on the following day. Then for twenty-eight days he absolutely abjured all food. He drank water, but that was all. Before going to bed he would take a pint of Apollinaris.

"Had he remained at his home in bed or taken perfect rest, his achievement would have been less remarkable. That is the course which always has been adopted by the professional fasters. Dr. Tanner, and the Italian, Succi, in their fasts were surrounded by attendants who allowed them scarcely to lift a hand, so that every ounce of energy might be conserved.

"Rathbun pursued a course diametrically opposite to this. He worked, and worked hard. He came down earlier to his office and went away later than usual. He made no effort to save himself. On the contrary, he seemed determined to make his task as hard as possible. On four of his fast days he spent the afternoons in a dentist's chair, at which times his nerves were tried as only dentists know how to do it.

"It was his idea to continue the fast until he began to feel hunger. After the first twenty-four hours his hunger disappeared, and he had no desire for food until the end of the fourth week, when the craving set in, and he immediately set about satisfying it in a moderate and careful manner. He consulted two physicians while the fast was going on, to see that he was suffering no injury that he could not appreciate himself. One was Dr. F. B. Carpenter, of Madison Avenue and thirty-eight Street, and the other, Dr. George J. Helmer, of Madison Avenue and Thirty-first Street. He saw Dr. Carpenter on the eighteenth and the twenty-first days, and Dr. Helmer on the twenty-fifth day. Both expressed surprise at his long fast and astonishment at his excellent condition.

"Mr. Rathbun is fifty-four years old, and five feet six inches in height. He does not look more than forty years old, and he is as active as a man of that age. He says he never felt better than when he was fasting, and that he has experienced no bad effects of any kind, while, on the other hand, he has reduced his weight to a normal limit and removed all danger of apoplexy.

"He got the idea of the fast from the new theory exploited by Dr. Edward Hooker Dewey, a practising physician of Meadville, Pa., who recommends fasting as a cure for many ailments, and advises all persons to go without breakfast and eat only two meals a day.

"'I became intensely interested in this new system,' said Mr. Rathbun yesterday, 'and I decided to put it to a practical test. Dr. Dewey had said that he had many patients fasting all the way from ten to thirty and forty days, and I concluded that if it did them so much good it would be just the thing for me. So I tried it.

"'On April 23 I ate my last meal, and from then until May 24 I had absolutely nothing to eat. I drank water, of course, for that is a matter of necessity. One cannot do without drink; but I took no nourishment. For the first twenty-four hours I was very hungry, and would have liked very much to take a square meal; but I resisted the temptation, and after the expiration of one day I had no desire to eat.

"'I had been in the habit of getting to my office about 8; now I get there at 7. I generally had left at 5.30; I now stayed until 6.30. I had been in the habit of taking an hour or an hour and a quarter for luncheon. The luncheon was now cut off, so I stayed in the office and worked. I sat there at my desk and put in a long, hard day's work, constantly writing.

"'At night I drank a bottle of Apollinaris, and went to bed at 8.30 and slept until 4 in the morning. I never enjoyed better sleep than in those four weeks. And I was in excellent condition as far as I could see in every other way. My mind was clear, my eye was sharper than usually, and all the functions were in excellent working order.

"'I had many amusing experiences. I went to a dentist on the first day. I had some work requiring several hours' labor on the part of the dentist. I said nothing to the doctor on the first day. Four or five days afterward I kept a second appointment with the dentist, and he asked me how the teeth worked which he had fixed before. I said to him: "I haven't tried them yet."

"'You can imagine the look of surprise on his face. When I told him that I was fasting, and had been since he had seen me before, he showed the greatest concern, and said he did not think I could go on with the dental work on account of the weakness of my nerves. He solicited me to go out and have just a bite of something. I refused, of course, and he continued the work. I visited him on two days after that until he had finished the work.

"'The men in my employ were greatly concerned about me, and thought I would break down. I used to weigh every night before leaving the office, and as they saw my constant wearing away they became more and more frightened, and finally appointed a committee to wait on me. The committee was headed by my manager, who begged me to eat. He brought along some fine ripe cherries to tempt me. I told him I would not eat them for one thousand dollars, for I was interested thoroughly in the fast by that time and would not have stopped.

"'After that they made no more attempts to stop the fast; but my friends all shook their heads, and said that when I started in to eat again I would find I was without a proper stomach.

"'On the twenty-eighth day the hunger began to come on again, and I began to eat under the advice of Dr. Carpenter. On the twenty-ninth day I drank a little bouillon, and afterward from day to day increased the amount of food to the normal. I suffered no inconvenience.'

"Mr. Rathbun says he is a firm believer in the no-breakfast system of hygiene advocated by Dr. Dewey, and that neither himself, his wife, nor any of the servants in his house eat breakfast, and as a result all are remarkably well. His two sons, one of whom was graduated at Harvard in 1896, and a second, who is still at Harvard, practise the no-breakfast system.

"Just before beginning his fast Mr. Rathbun ordered a suit of clothes at his tailor's. He did not go for it until the end of his long fast. Being something of a practical joker, besides a man of great nerve, he walked into the tailor-shop and let the tailor try his new suit on to see if it was all right.

"When he slipped on the coat the tailor stood aghast. There was apparently the same man he had measured twenty-eight days previously standing before him in perfect health, but as to dimensions not at all the same man.

"'It doesn't fit any part of you,' said the tailor, after the suit had been tried on. In the tailor's book Rathbun's measurement was entered: 'Forty-three inches around the waist and forty-two around the chest.' When he went for his suit his measurements were thirty-eight around the waist and thirty-eight around the chest.

"Dr. Dewey's theory, which led Rathbun to make his long fast, is that the brain is the centre of every mind and muscle energy, a sort of self-charging dynamo, with the heart, lungs, and all the other parts only as so many machines to be run by it; that the brain has the power of feeding itself on the less important parts of the body without loss of its own structure, and that as the operation of digestion is a tax on the brain, a long period of fasting gives the brain a rest, by which means the brain is able to build itself up, which means the upbuilding of the whole body.

"In this way, it is asserted, the alcohol habit is cured and other diseases eradicated.

"Dr. F. B. Carpenter said yesterday to a reporter for *The Press* that he had not recommended Mr. Rathbun to take the fast, but had advised him while it was going on and after it was over. The doctor said he was inclined to believe there might be something in the no-breakfast system, as a great many persons eat and drink altogether too much.

"Dr. Helmer said he had examined Rathbun on the twenty-fifth day, and had found him in surprisingly good condition."

Mr. Rathbun had been on the no-breakfast plan for several years, and he was one of the first to write me after my book came out. It was not without reason he feared apoplexy, for Ex-Gov. Flower, an over-weighted man, had gone down to instant death though seemingly in perfect health and in the prime of business energy and mental capacity. During his fast my only trouble with him was in his drinking so much water without thirst, thus greatly and needlessly adding to the work of the kidneys.

Mr. Rathbun was so disappointed over the skepticism of New York physicians as to the reliability of the fast that he determined to undergo a longer one under such surveillance as would enforce conviction. He was mainly actuated, however, to go through the ordeal in the interests of science.

Again I had trouble with him on the water question, wishing him to drink only as thirst incited. He was differently advised by an eminent Boston physician, who, taking a great interest in the case, wrote him that he should have great care to drink certain definite amounts for the necessary fluidity of the blood. I had to respond that thirst would duly indicate this need; that in my cases of protracted fasts from acute sicknesses not one had been advised to take even a teaspoonful of water for such reasons; that at the closing days before recovery of such cases there was only the least desire for water, and this with no indication of need from the blood. Mr. Rathbun did not escape some trouble from overworked kidneys, and he became convinced that my theory and practice were more in line with physiology.

This fast was made a matter of daily record by the leading New York journals, and he became such a subject of general interest that in addition to his ordinary business he was greatly overtaxed, and was compelled to give up the fast on the thirty-fifth day, in part from the exhaustion of over-excitement.

This case was summed up as follows by the *New York Press*, February 27, 1900:

"Milton Rathbun has ended his long fast.

"After thirty-five days, in which solid food or any liquid other than water was a stranger to his palate, he became extremely hungry on Sunday night. At first he resisted the longing to eat and tried to sleep it off. But he awoke in a few hours hungrier than ever, and then he decided he had fasted as long as was good for him.

"He ate a modest, light meal and went back to bed, only to awake still hungry. Then he ate an orange, and was asleep again in a jiffy. A bowl of milk and cream and crackers sufficed for his breakfast, and at noon yesterday he enjoyed his first hearty meal.

"As he walked around the parlor of his home in Mount Vernon, lighter by forty-three pounds than he was on January 21, this man of fifty-five years and iron will said:

"'I feel like a boy again. I think I could vault over a six-foot fence.'

"Mrs. Rathbun herself knows what it is to fast. For five years such a thing as breakfast has been an unknown quantity in her house, save when guests were present or for the servants. To this abstinence Mrs. Rathbun attributes the curing of catarrh, from which she had suffered previously. And as she and her husband do, so do their two sons.

"After the first few days of abstinence he had felt no desire to eat until Sunday evening. Then he became hungry—ravenously so. His first fast of a year ago—it was twenty-eight days then—had taught him that sleep took away the longing for food, and, too, he had said he would make his fast last forty days this time. So he went to bed and to sleep.

"But he awoke at 11 o'clock; he was hungrier than ever, and he decided not to resist his inclination for food. Calling his wife he asked her for an orange, and ate it; then he took another. His next demand was for oysters, and a dozen large, juicy ones disappeared rapidly, to the accompaniment of five soda crackers. Then he drank about two-thirds of a cup of beef-tea, and some Oolong tea. His appetite was not sated by any means, but he knew the danger of overloading his stomach, so he stopped.

"He soon was slumbering again, but he was wide awake at 2 o'clock in the morning. And his hunger was with him still. He ate an orange to appease the craving, and again sought his pillow. He slept again until 6 o'clock, and then, breaking some crackers in a bowl of milk and cream, he ate again.

"At noon a meal was served to the still hungry man. He began with a little clam-broth; then came half a dozen steamed clams, followed by a small portion of mock-turtle soup. Of a squab he ate one-half, and with it some canned pease and fried potatoes; while for dessert he had a little lemon ice.

"'That was good,' he exclaimed, as he finished. The remark was unnecessary; the relish with which he had eaten was convincing testimony of his enjoyment. Asked why he had decided not to fast for the full forty days, he said:

"'I ate just because I was hungry.'

"Asked how the weather affected him, he said:

"'When I began there was a spell of cold weather, and I found it rather hard to keep warm at night. But it soon passed away, and I made it a point to wear the same underclothing and outer garments as usual. Oh, yes; I did wear a different pair of trousers. I had them made five years ago, but they were so tight around the waist I could never wear them. They are as loose as can be now, however.'

"'From a scientific standpoint,' said Professor R. Ogden Doremus yesterday, 'it is the most interesting and valuable experiment I have known. Mr. Rathbun is a man of great nerve force. The very fact that he attended to his business was what saved him, in keeping his mind away from the thought of food. He could not have done it had he been on exhibition or if he had remained at home. If he had been at sea, in an open boat, he could not have lasted more than ten days. He would have had nothing to think of but his hunger.'

"Dr. George J. Helmer, who has given no little attention to Mr. Rathbun, said:

"'I have examined him several times; I did so when his thirty days were up. Well, it was remarkable. It's a wonderful exhibition, that will attract the attention of the medical world. His heart is as clear as a bell and his kidneys are perfect. He is in absolutely rugged health. His temperature was normal, his eye clear, and to-day, upon examination, any insurance company would rate him as an A1 risk.'

"Following is from the diary kept during his fast, and furnished by Milton Rathbun to *The Press*:

"*First Day*, Jan. 22, 8.45 A. M.—Weight, 207 pounds; height, 5 ft. $6\frac{1}{2}$ inches; chest measure, $43\frac{1}{2}$ inches; waist measure, $43\frac{1}{2}$ inches; hip measure, $46\frac{1}{2}$ inches; calf measure, 17 inches; biceps measure, 14 inches; forearm, 12 inches. 3 P. M., feels well, but hungry. In the evening felt well, not being hungry or thirsty. Have taken no water.

"*Tuesday*, Jan. 23.—Slept well until 6 A. M. Rested a while, then took sponge bath and rubdown. At 8.45 weighed 200 pounds. Feel good, but a little weak. 12 o'clock M., no appetite and feverish. 4 P. M., weighed 199 pounds; went home; drank one pint of water during the evening.

"*Wednesday*, Jan. 24.—Slept well for nine hours. Got up at 6 A. M., drank one glass of water and took train to the city. 8.30 A. M., weighed $198\frac{1}{2}$ pounds; only half pound lost, which shows how greedily the tissues absorb moisture and add to weight. 12 o'clock M., have no appetite nor thirst, and no fever. Retired at 9 o'clock, feeling comfortable but a little feverish.

"*Thursday*, Jan. 25.—After having slept seven and one-half hours took a sponge bath and brisk rubdown. Came to the city, and at 8.25 A. M. weighed 195 pounds. Feeling good, with no fever nor appetite. 4.45 P. M., weighed

193 pounds. At home during the evening drank two and one-half glasses of water.

"*Friday*, Jan. 26.—Slept eight hours. No appetite and feeling stronger. Examined by Professor Doremus and Dr. Carpenter. Retired at 9 o'clock, feeling first class.

"*Saturday*, Jan. 27.—Came to the city on the 7.45 A. M. train. Weighed 191 pounds. Feeling good. No fever and no appetite.

"*Sunday*, Jan. 28.—Drank one glass of water when I got up. During the day and evening drank three more glasses of water. Retired feeling first class.

"*Monday*, Jan. 29.—Slept eight hours last night, and came to the city on the 7.45 A. M. train. At 8.25 weighed 189 pounds. 4 P. M., was examined by Dr. F. B. Carpenter, who found the temperature $98\frac{1}{2}°$ F., pulse regular, tongue clean. Measurements were: waist, 41 inches; chest, 41 inches; hip, 45 inches; calf, 16 inches; biceps, $13\frac{1}{2}$ inches; forearm, $11\frac{1}{2}$ inches. 5.15 P. M., weighed 188 pounds.

"*Tuesday*, Jan. 30.—Slept eight hours; weighed 188 pounds, same as the night before; feeling good. 5.30 P. M., weighed $185\frac{1}{2}$ pounds.

"*Wednesday*, Jan. 31.—Slept $7\frac{1}{2}$ hours, drank one and one-half glasses of water; weighed at 8.25 A. M. 187 pounds; Dr. Carpenter found temperature 98° F., and pulse 88; Professor Doremus called a little later; weighed $184\frac{1}{2}$ pounds.

"*Thursday*, Feb. 1.—Rested quietly when not asleep; drank only one and three-quarters glasses of water all day; weighed 184 pounds; retired feeling good.

"*Friday*, Feb. 2.—Not feeling any hunger; was examined by F. B. Carpenter; temperature, 98° F.; pulse, 84; weighed 183 pounds; retired feeling well, but tired.

"*Saturday*, Feb. 3.—Somewhat wakeful during the night. 5.45 P. M., weighed 182 pounds.

"*Sunday*, Feb. 4.—Read all day and felt well.

"*Monday*, Feb. 5.—2 P. M., temperature, 98.4° F.; pulse, 82; tongue clean. Measurements were: waist, 41 inches; chest, 41 inches; hip, 43 inches; calf, 14½ inches; biceps, 13½ inches; forearm, 11½ inches; went to bed feeling a trifle feverish.

"*Tuesday*, Feb. 6.—Wakeful during the night. 11 A. M., had my eyes examined by Dr. L. H. Matthez, oculist, and found a marked improvement in my sight over same tests of two months previous, being 7 degrees stronger; felt a little weak, but no fever or appetite; weighed 180 pounds; feeling somewhat exhausted from the day's labor and in entertaining guests.

"*Wednesday*, Feb. 7.—Slept about seven hours during the night; when I awoke felt rested; temperature, 98.2° F.; pulse, 80; have felt well all day; went to bed at 9.30; some fever.

"*Thursday*, Feb. 8.—Woke up two or three times during the night. Drank water during the night and first thing this morning when I got up. Came to the city, and at 9 o'clock weighed 182 pounds, showing a gain of two pounds over last night. Not feeling so well owing to the amount of water I drank last night, which was induced by feverishness.

"*Friday*, Feb. 9.—Feeling first rate. At 8.25 A. M. weighed 180 pounds. Heart action normal. No enlargement of the spleen or liver.

"*Saturday*, Feb. 10.—Lost nothing in weight during the day and have felt well all the while.

"*Sunday*, Feb. 11.—Passed the day in reading and drank frequently of water.

"*Monday*, Feb. 12.—This being a holiday, did not go to the city. Passed the day in entertaining callers. Have not felt quite so well owing to a slight cold settling in my left kidney.

"*Tuesday*, Feb. 13.—Measurements: waist, 38½ inches; chest, 40 inches; hip, 43 inches; calf, 14½ inches; biceps, 12½ inches; forearm, 11 inches; weight, 177½ pounds.

"*Wednesday*, Feb. 14.—I attribute the cause of loss of sleep to a hard day's work and in reading too long last evening.

"*Thursday*, Feb. 15.—Somewhat wakeful during the night. Retired at 7.30 o'clock, after a hard day's work.

"*Friday*, Feb. 16.—3.30 P. M., temperature, 98.5° F.; pulse, 74; tongue clean; weighed $172\frac{1}{2}$ pounds. During the evening drank one cup of hot water.

"*Saturday*, Feb. 17.—After a restful night felt well all day.

"*Sunday*, Feb. 18.—Retired at 9 o'clock and have rested a good deal during the day.

"*Monday*, Feb. 19.—Weighed $169\frac{1}{2}$ pounds, and retired feeling well.

"*Tuesday*, Feb. 20.—Weighed $168\frac{1}{2}$ pounds; was examined by Dr. Helmer, who found me in excellent condition; 4.30 P. M., weighed $169\frac{1}{2}$ pounds, a gain of one pound during the day, on account of drinking a little more water than usual.

"*Wednesday*, Feb. 21.—Temperature, 98.5° F.; pulse, 69; 4 P. M., weighed $168\frac{1}{2}$ pounds; have not felt quite so well during the day.

"*Thursday*, Feb. 22.—Occupied the day—holiday—in reading and reclining, and went to bed feeling pretty well.

"*Friday*, Feb. 23.—At 8.30 A. M. weighed 166 pounds; 3.30 P. M., temperature, 99° F.; pulse, 98; lung expansion, $2\frac{3}{4}$ inches; went home and to bed, feeling considerably exhausted owing to a hard day's work and too many callers.

"*Saturday*, Feb. 24.—Did not rest very well from overtaxing the brain yesterday. Do not feel quite so well this morning owing to that fact and from drinking too much water during the past twenty-four hours. At 8.25 A. M. weighed 166 pounds; went home not feeling well to-day on account of some stomach disturbance, which probably comes from drinking too much water; did not drink any water during the evening; feeling quite tired at bedtime.

"*Sunday*, Feb. 25.—Slept nine hours and rested well, and did not drink any water during the night. Kept quiet all day, lying down most of the time, and felt the coming of hunger about 6 o'clock.

12 o'clock noon, pulse regular; tongue clean; temperature, 98.2°F.; weighed 164 pounds. Measurements were: waist, $36\frac{1}{2}$ inches; chest, 38 inches; hip, $40\frac{1}{2}$ inches; calf, 14 inches; biceps, 11 inches; forearm, 10 inches.

Was in bed at 8 o'clock, still feeling hungry, and after a short sleep woke up at 11 o'clock with a sharp appetite, and ate a dozen raw oysters, two oranges, two-thirds cup of beef-tea, five crackers, and part of a cup of Oolong tea.

I insert a photograph of Mr. Rathbun taken shortly after his second fast. There had been five years' trial of the No-Breakfast Plan before these fasting demonstrations.

One of the hardest things on earth as a mental operation is to be fair to the opposition. Now lest I have beguiled my readers overmuch by the force of my convictions even to the point of danger, I will give an estimate of the danger of fasting by one of the most eminent physicians of New York City, Dr. George F. Shrady. I quote from an interview reported in the New York *Sun*:

"The strange case of Milton Rathbun, of Mt. Vernon, who, to reduce his flesh and generally tone up his system, is said to have gone without food of any sort for thirty-six days, still continues to be the subject of more or less discussion among the medical men of the city. Dr. George F. Shrady, in speaking last evening of Mr. Rathbun's remarkable exploit, said:

"'There are three things to say about it. In the first place, the fact, if it be a fact, as it seems to be, is astonishing; secondly, it was very foolish; and thirdly, it would be a very unfortunate and dangerous thing to popularize such experiments. Now as to whether the gentleman in question actually did go thirty-six days without taking nourishment of any sort is a matter I will not discuss. If he were a professional faster, I would hardly hesitate to say his claim was fraudulent, for I am fully convinced that all the professional fasters are frauds. They are simply adept sleight-of-hand men. They work out some adroit trick by which they may get nourishment into their systems in spite of the always more or less negligent or suspicious watchers, and then advertise for a forty days' or sixty days' 'fast.'

"'Now, mind you, I do not say this Mt. Vernon case is anything of this sort. I only say that if it is true it is most astounding. It is in flat contradiction of all the authorities on the subject of a human being's ability to do without food. The extreme limit of all well-authenticated cases of total abstinence from nourishment is from nine to ten days. Imprisoned miners have been known to go that time and survive.

"'But at all events it was a very foolish thing for Mr. Rathbun to do. About that there can be no manner of doubt. What will be the future effect upon him—upon his heart action, upon his impoverished blood, upon his nervous system, upon his organs of nutrition, necessarily paralyzed for days? These are grave questions, the answers to which may be unpleasant to Mr. Rathbun as they reveal themselves to him in the future. You cannot fly in the face of Nature and ignore all her laws in that way with impunity. She exacts her penalties and there is no court of appeals in her realm.

"'When I say that the extreme limits of abstinence from nourishment in clearly authenticated cases is from nine to ten days, you must not get the impression that all persons can last that long.

"'It is a question of environment, of mental condition—whether buoyed by hope or stimulated by ambition to do a great feat—and above all, of course, of the physical condition of the faster. Without food the body absorbs its own tissues. Mr. Rathbun, I am told, was a very heavy man with a superabundance of tissue. Naturally he could go longer without nourishment than a weak, attenuated, thin-blooded man.

"'Yet Mr. Rathbun was exercising daily and about his usual avocations, and he abstained from food for thirty-six days! Well, it's remarkable!

"'But I sincerely hope Mr. Rathbun will have no imitators. It would be a very unfortunate thing, fraught with grave possibilities, if the newspaper accounts of his reduction in weight and general improvement in health were to move others to follow his example. Many persons would be injured for life, physically wrecked, and perhaps actually killed if they conscientiously did the fifth part of what he is said to have done.

"'And right here it may be said that there is a great deal of exaggeration in the sweeping statements made about people eating too much. If a man sleeps well, goes about his business in a cheerful frame of mind, and does not get what is called "out-of-sorts," he may be pretty sure he is not eating too much, even though he eat a good deal. My observation is that the average man who works and gets a proper amount of exercise does not eat too much. If you want to get work done by the engine, you have got to stoke up the furnace. If a man wants to keep his vital energies up to par he has got to put in the fuel—that is, the food.

"'Of course, there are those who lead sedentary lives who get too much absorbed in the pleasures of the table and overfeed. There are a sufficient number of these, to be sure, but I think they are the exception. But it will be a sad mistake if even they seek a road to health by Mr. Rathbun's starvation methods.'"

The doctor is astonished, and so am I that he is astonished. This would seem to imply that he has never had cases of acute sickness in which the amount of food taken during many days or even weeks was too small to play any part as a life-prolonging factor.

"It was a foolish, even dangerous experiment." How foolish or dangerous? What vital organs suffered? Was there evidence of a loss of anything but fat? What organs were "necessarily paralyzed" during the fast? Evidently not the brain, else longer days of labor would not have been possible; and the grave future possibilities in heart action, impoverished blood, nervous system, upon organs of nutrition "necessarily paralyzed" for days; and the extreme limit of nine or ten days before death from starvation; and that without food the *body* lives on its own tissues!

One can easily see that the earnest doctor is full of strong impressions that have little of the flavor of science: truth that is not self-evident should have the instant logic in easy reach. I may here say that my hygienic scheme has from the first been subject to similar attacks by physicians from the standpoint of impressions, but no physician has ventured into print against it after becoming aware of its physiologic basis.

I am happy to assure all readers that in all the involuntary fasts of my cases of acute sickness or in the voluntary fasts in chronic disease, has there been any other than improved general health as the result. Notably was this the case in a man who fasted ten years ago for forty days for an ulcer of the stomach, and who had been troubled with indigestion for more than forty years. He had become nearly a mental and physical wreck when he took to his bed with an abolished appetite. There have since been some ten years of nearly perfect health, and now in his seventy-seventh year he is the youngest-looking man for his age I have ever seen. He walks the streets with the gait of a youth of twenty. To do without food without hunger does not tax any vital power, as Dr. Shrady may yet become aware.

The next fast to have a brief notoriety as the "most remarkable on record" occurred in Philadelphia, the medical center of America, and beneath the very shadow of its great medical schools; in Philadelphia, a city that surpasses all other cities for the wisest conservatism, for all-around level-headedness. Its journals are rarely equalled for their clean, winnowed columns; there is no "yellow" journalism in that great, fair city, known as the "Quaker City."

Miss Estella Kuenzel, a lady of twenty-two years, of acutest, finest sensibilities, born to live in June and not in March, lost her mental health to a degree that death became the final object of desire.

She had a friend in a bright young man of the name of Henry Ritter, chemist and photographer at the Drexel Institute, a born scientist, and who possesses the very genius of the pains and persistence of science. Well versed in the science of the morning fast, he believed that a fast which would merely end with hunger would result in all-around improvement. A fast was instituted which he thought would not last more than a few days, but went on until the days merged into weeks: it went on because only general improvement attended it.

I first heard of it in a letter written by him on the thirty-eighth day of the fast, during which there had been a walk of seven miles. On the forty-second day of the fast I had a brief letter from Miss K., in which every line was radiant with cheer.

At the Asylum five feedings per day were ordered, and at first were rejected; but finally she accepted them as a means to end her unhappy life; took them in bed, and in the last weeks seemed to be fleshing up, as there was a gain of seventeen pounds above the normal, of water—she had become dropsical. The last professional expert in her case advised a half-gallon of milk daily in addition to the three regular meals—making a five-meal plan.

To carry out an unopposed fast it was necessary to take her to a home where the parents would be ignorant of this radical means to a cure.

The following is from Mr. Ritter's letters:

"I had made my views known to the parents and daughter when the case commenced, and after the failure of these methods they decided to let me have charge of the case, which was on Sept. 30, 1899. I at once requested them to send her to the house of some friends to whom I made my views known. We then discharged the nurse who had gone with her. With doctor and nurse gone there was free room for Nature's victory (the young lady being as deeply interested as any). We put her upon the rest, which was the only needed sign since her first signs of breakdown appeared Oct. 2, at the supper table, being the last meal she has taken up to to-day, Nov. 9, this being, as you will see, the thirty-eighth day of her fast, with cheerfulness and strength holding full sway. I put her to bed on the first day, to which she kept, with an occasional day in the rocker, until the eleventh day, when she took a walk of about one mile. Then she rested indoors until the twentieth day, when we went to church, walking a little over two miles, with no fatigue or tired feelings. I forgot to mention that we had been out driving in the bracing air for over three hours in the afternoon. On the twenty-first and twenty-second days, indoors, walking and working around the house, reading, etc. On the twenty-third day walked through the country for three miles, stopping at friends to enlighten them upon 'Nature's Laws;' twenty-fourth day, eight miles, no fatigue; twenty-fifth day, between seven and eight miles, no fatigue; twenty-sixth day, walked one and a half hours; twenty-ninth day, rainy, no walks; thirtieth day, walked in the evening for two and a half hours; thirty-first day, walked seven miles, no fatigue; thirty-second day, rainy, no walks; thirty-third day, went to the Exposition, walked all day from 2 P. M. until 11.30 P. M. (with rest while at the performance we attended of not over one and a quarter hours), this being the only resting, possibly two hours, during the whole time.

"Weight taken at the start, one hundred and forty pounds; at the Exposition one hundred and twenty-five and three-quarters pounds; no sense of tired feeling, but hunger started to assert itself for a period of about three hours, after which it passed over.

"On the thirty-fourth day went driving; thirty-fifth day, walked one mile, then went to the asylum to show the results. The physicians in charge were simply astounded, and would hardly believe it possible for one to be so active while taking no food. I believe we have done quite a little good there, as they have expressed the desire to try the same on others. They examined the tongue and took the pulse, finding both in good, normal state; in the evening walked another mile, visiting the other doctors whom her parents called in. On the thirty-sixth day walked one and a half miles; thirty-seventh day, walked seven miles, hunger sensation becoming decided.

"I have given you a sketch of this case because it seems to me an unusual one owing to the great activity."

"November 18, 1899.

"Miss Kuenzel's hunger arrived as per Nature's demand on the forty-fifth day at noon. One poached egg and two slices of toast (whole wheat). There was an intense relish for her simple fare, but not the least sign or desire for haste in eating. She was amply satisfied for the day, and relished the same bill of fare and quantity for the forty-sixth day, with a very slight luncheon in the evening. We had been to the Exposition the night of the forty-fourth day, when the tongue again started cleaning and a most distinct craving for food presented itself. It persisted on retiring, and also on the next morning, when she felt that Nature again was ready for her wonderful chemistry of digestion. I had her weight taken after her first meal, which revealed a loss of twenty pounds. We called to see the professor under whom she was last placed, and he was surprised with the clearness of her mental condition and good general appearance, though he observed she had gotten a trifle thinner, but which he had also in view to accomplish upon a five-meal plan per day. He tried his best to confuse and trouble her with questions, etc., but found her too intensely awake, and she won the victory by cornering him in his own set traps. We received his congratulations and were made to promise to call again. I have now been with her to seven physicians who were interested, and have shown them Nature's own unhampered work.

"Miss Kuenzel has now an intense desire to help others. You are at liberty to make use of Nature's work in her case for the benefit of others, and I shall be only too glad to give you any desired information that may be of use. The good work you have started will, I am sure, never end; and it will prove a pleasure to me indeed to work with added interest for the benefit of those in need of the same in the future."

The forty-fourth day of the fast was the busiest of all with her. She arose at 8.30 A. M. to attend to her affairs until the late afternoon, when she and her friend met a sister, by appointment from her home, at the Exposition. Several hours were spent there, and when they took the street car for return the only vacant seat was accepted by the sister, because she was tired, and not knowing that there were forty-four days without food with her sister, who was not tired. A striking feature of these daily walks was that they did not cause marked fatigue. Miss Kuenzel retired near midnight without unusual fatigue, and so ended the forty-fourth day of the fast.

I quote from the *Chester County Times* of Feb. 12, 1899:

"'Conclusive evidence is being multiplied as to the wonderful power of fasting in the restoration of health, but it is only more recently that its power in the case of insanity is even yet more wonderful. A recent case is as near home as the city of Philadelphia, and those interested are very willing that others may know of it, so that its usefulness may be extended and its value appreciated. The discovery was made by Dr. E. H. Dewey, of Meadville, Pa., and tidings of the good work are being spread by Charles C. Haskell & Son, of Norwich, Conn. The editor of this paper knows somewhat the value of the discovery by an experience of several years. We give a letter from the lady who was cured.

"'PHILADELPHIA, PA., Dec. 12, 1899.

"'*My Dear Mr. Haskell:*

"'I have received your letter of the 9th inst., and at last find time to fulfil the request for a statement. In regard to my *wonderful cure* through "The New Gospel of Health," I would state that the second week after Christmas, 1898, I first had a paralyzing effect which affected the right side of face, body, and limbs, also tongue, which nearly prevented my speaking. This passed over and I again began working at my position as milliner in a large establishment, and after a short while became so dizzy and confused that I was compelled to ask my friends to direct me home. (This was around Easter, 1899.) I was then taken to a doctor, who at once requested me to stop working, and to take a *complete rest*, but not for the stomach, as he prescribed a severe and exacting master to stimulate the *tired and overworked stomach* to *renewed life*, and so give the nerves plenty of pure food, as they were in need of same. I then, after getting a ravenous hunger, weakened myself still more and became worse. My stomach felt numb and paralyzed, as did also my other internal organs, but this was put down against me as an illusion. So a *professor of nervous diseases* was called in consultation, owing to my many desires to die (as life had no sunshine, flowers, or music for me); I was simply living a living death of torture which these professors would have were illusions. My parents were then informed that I must be sent to an asylum, where I was for ten long weeks. *They* also told me that my feelings were illusions, and proceeded to banish the same by giving the *tired-out nerves a little rest* and *plenty of nourishment* on a *five-meal* plan per day. If refused (owing to a loss of appetite), I was threatened to have nature helped by the aid of a stomach or nasal tube. I lost none of my illusions while there, as I could not feel any improvement in my feelings. I left the institution June 28, 1899, feeling no better; in fact, worse than when I arrived there. I was then taken from one doctor to another, the one wishing to operate, the other not; one advising me to go to the seashore, country, etc., but *none* to give my stomach the needed vacation.

"'It was then that my friend, Mr. Ritter, stepped in, as he saw the failures of professors and specialists, and begged my parents to let him have a chance to demonstrate what Dr. Dewey's method would do for melancholy illusions and tired-out stomachs and nerves. I then went to friends, and, in entire ignorance of my parents, began under directions of Mr. Ritter the most natural, sensible, and cheapest of all cures. I began my fast on Oct. 3, and broke the same on Nov. 16. During the first week of my fast I was in bed; during the second (excepting the eleventh day, when I took my first walk of seven-eighths of a mile) I was in bed, in rocker, reading, etc. On the twentieth day, after a drive of three hours, went to church, walking two and one-sixteenth miles. I then stayed indoors again on the twenty-first and twenty-second days, and then started taking daily walks (weather permitting). I went out walking twenty-three out of the forty-five days of my fast, and during that time walked one hundred and twelve miles. This was besides the carriage-drives, Exposition, and evening gatherings (walking to same included). I did not in the least feel tired or weak, but happier and brighter each day of the fast, as I could feel the effects of a new life throughout my whole body. My mind also became clearer and dizziness became a thing of the past. This was indeed *joy supreme to me*, and life became once more a joy instead of a burden. Sunshine, trees, flowers, etc., again made an impression, and my parents, sisters, and friends are rejoiced to see me in my happy normal state of health.

"'I have gone through a year of unspeakable torture brought on by overwork and *human-wise professors*; but at last, through the wonderful teachings Dr. Dewey has given to mankind, and through a friend, who was able to preach the "New Gospel of Health," am now well, strong, and happy. May God only help and bless the many sufferers throughout the world (especially in the asylums) with the rays of this Gospel. I have been saved, no doubt, from a gloomy future, and may such be the realization of many more unfortunate souls is the sincere wish through experience of

     "'Yours very sincerely,
      "'ESTELLA F. KUENZEL.'"

This case was summed up in the Philadelphia *Public Ledger* of Dec. 25, 1899, whose columns are guarded with unsurpassed care, as follows:

"One of those cases which a judicious editor ponders in no little perplexity is that of a young lady who was taken out of an insane hospital and subjected to a protracted fast, without medical supervision, and with results that appear to have been quite successful. On the one hand, there is the benefit that may be derived by having the attention of the profession called to the subject, with possibly good results; on the other hand, there is the danger of having a lot of ignorant or impulsive people risking their lives by starving themselves for this or that real or fancied disease, forgetting the adage that a little knowledge is a dangerous thing, especially in therapeutics.

"The mind of the young lady referred to became affected about a year ago, and after what was regarded by her parents as an unprofitable period of treatment for two and a half months in a hospital for the insane she has been apparently cured by fasting—some would call it starvation. The case has been attracting attention and discussion lately in a growing circle that has included a few physicians.

"The subject is a Miss K., aged twenty-two years. Henry Ritter, who has charge of the Photography Department of the Drexel Institute, and who is better acquainted with the matter than any one else, furnished a *Ledger* reporter with the particulars as they are here given, the name and address of the young lady, for obvious reasons, being omitted. Mr. Ritter was at first loath to have any publicity given the case, but felt upon reflection that the results were properly a subject matter for inquiry by physicians, at least, not to speak of others who may be interested.

"Miss K., by the advice of specialists who had treated her at home, was put under treatment for melancholy in an institution for the insane. Mr. Ritter, being an intimate friend of the family, visited her, and, he says, found her retrograding. She was receiving three meals a day, with two luncheons between them. Having built up his own digestive powers by following the tenets laid down by Dr. Dewey, a Crawford county physician, he had become a student and advocate of the latter's theory, briefly stated, that no food should be given to a patient except in response to a natural call or appetite for it. Believing that no improvement could result from the course Miss K. was receiving in the hospital, he prevailed upon her parents to permit him to have her placed in the home of a friend, and suggested the fasting process. This was the more readily done as the physicians in whose care she had been advised her parents to leave their daughter as much as possible among strangers.

"This young lady, according to Mr. Ritter, was absolutely without food for forty-five days, beginning October 3 and ending November 16. He says he did not fear, as others did, that she would starve, as the authority he depended on had never fed a sick patient during a practice covering twenty-two years, no matter how protracted the case might have been, and claimed to have had only the best results. 'This,' said Mr. Ritter, 'is on the theory that, since all bodily energy is the result of the brain, by abstaining from feeding in the absence of appetite there is all the energy of cure undiverted by needless waste in the stomach. Feeding the sick, this physician contends, is a tax on their vital power, adding indigestion to whatever other troubles exist: because the brain has the power in sickness to absorb nourishment from the body, as predigested food, so that it never loses weight, even in death from starvation.'

"The patient herself became interested, Mr. Ritter says, and evidenced great relief from abstinence from enforced periodic feeding. Gradually a numb feeling of which she had complained as affecting her internal organs, and which had been ascribed to her illusions, left her, and she appeared to gain daily in strength and brightness. Mr. Ritter's narrative proceeds:

"'On the eleventh day of her fast a walk was suggested, and she covered about seven-eighths of a mile; on the twentieth day she was taken for a carriage drive of three hours in the afternoon, and in the evening she walked to church and back, a distance of something more than two miles. From the twenty-third day she took walks daily, excepting on October 31 and November 3, when rain prevented. She visited friends and the theatre and the Exposition, went to church several times, to the hospital where she had been a patient—this on the thirty-fifth day of her fast—and to the Drexel Institute on the thirty-ninth and forty-second days. A table of dates shows that she walked from two or three to six and eight and as high as nine miles a day during the period of forty-five days that she abstained from food, with a general increase of strength and cheer and no sign of fatigue. Hunger sensations were marked on the forty-fourth day and night, and on the morning of the forty-fifth day Miss K. broke the fast by eating a poached egg and two slices of buttered whole wheat toasted bread.

"'During her fast she was seen by seven physicians and medical professors, President MacAlister and professors of the Drexel Institute, and many others.'

"The young lady's weight at the beginning of the fast, Mr. Ritter says, was one hundred and forty pounds, and just after the meal with which she broke the fast she weighed one hundred and twenty pounds. By December 15 she had regained nine pounds, meanwhile eating one meal daily and sometimes two, with an occasional light luncheon.

"Dr. Chase, medical director of the institution above referred to, was visited on Saturday by a *Ledger* reporter in regard to the case of Miss K. He had been informed of her long fast and of its results, and had seen Miss K. herself when she called at the asylum on the thirty-fifth day of the fast. He said that when she was first brought to the asylum she was suffering from melancholia, and was put under the treatment which all the leading alienists had found most beneficial for persons suffering from nervous disorders, viz., quiet, rest of mind and body, and full, nourishing diet, carefully selected to produce the best results. During the time she remained at the asylum she improved both in bodily and mental health.

"Referring to the treatment she had received under Mr. Ritter's supervision since leaving the asylum, Dr. Chase said he had first heard of the system through a work published two years ago by Dr. George S. Keith, of London, from which he first learned of Dr. Dewey, who also uses the fasting cure. In all the cases cited by Dr. Keith none had been afflicted with any mental disorder. He looked upon the cases, however, as showing some remarkable results, warranting a careful study. But it would not do to adopt such a system without a most thorough examination. As 'one swallow does not make a summer,' neither will one case nor half a dozen cases cured by such a method prove anything. No universal method can be adopted for treating disease. Hardly two cases are alike. Cures also may be brought about in different ways if the exact condition of the patient is understood.

"'Mr. Ritter says the patient lent herself very willingly to the treatment, which was a great deal to start out with in her case. But I am surprised that a young man with no medical knowledge would do a thing like that. The treatment might easily have resulted differently. If he had been a doctor, he would have had that fact to sustain him in case he got into trouble. The case might very well have resulted fatally, because the treatment was so contrary to what would naturally be pursued by physicians in nervous cases.

"'I do not ridicule the system. There have been cases which were cured by ways not recognized by the general practitioner after they had been given up. I am a firm believer that in selected cases the fasting method would be efficacious, but I do not believe in its general application.

"'Mr. Ritter is evidently an enthusiast, and apt to overstate the points in favor of the method, neglecting those which tell against it. It is too early yet to say what the outcome of Miss K.'s case will be. I think the matter ought to be looked into more fully. Mr. Ritter could not have been with the patient at all times. It is a remarkable thing that she should have kept up and had the strength reported, unless she had some food. He may have been deceived in that.'"

During several months since the fast there have been the best physical *health* and mental condition, the weight having increased several pounds above the former average.

Mr. Ritter conducted this case in a blaze of publicity. He showed it to no less than seven physicians, some of whom were college professors, and one of them at near the close of the fast suggested that if food were not soon taken a sudden collapse would be the result. There seemed to have been less danger of this calamity on the forty-fourth day than on any other.

The reliability of the fast was so clearly evident that the leading papers of the city accepted it as authentic news and of the most startling kind. *The*

Times gave several columns of its first page to an illustrated article.[1]

The accompanying illustration shows Miss Kuenzel on the forty-first day of her fast. She walked seven miles on this day without any signs of fatigue.

MISS ESTELLA F. KUENZEL, FORTY-FIRST DAY OF FAST.

The following table of miles walked were measured from exact diary notes with bicycle and cyclometer after the fast was broken. The table gives the total sum of each day, walks being taken both afternoon and evenings of same day.

Date.	Miles.
October 3	

"	4	
"	5	
"	6	
"	7	
"	8	
"	9	
"	10	
"	11	
"	12	
"	13	$7/8$
"	14	
"	15	
"	16	
"	17	
"	18	
"	19	
"	20	
"	21	
"	22	$2\,1/16$
"	23	
"	24	
"	25	3
"	26	$6\,5/8$
"	27	$5\,7/8$
"	28	$4\,1/2$
"	29	$4\,1/8$
"	30	$5\,5/8$
"	31	rain
November	1	$6\,3/4$
"	2	8
"	3	rain
"	4	9

"	5	6
"	6	3¾
"	7	1½
"	8	7¼
"	9	7
"	10	4¼
"	11	2⅝
"	12	7
"	13	2¼
"	14	3¼
"	15	5
"	16	5¾
		112¹⁄₁₆

The next fast, under the care of Mr. Ritter, still holds the record as being the most remarkable for its number of days and the miracle of results. The following account of it appeared in the *North American*, one of whose editors had personal knowledge of its history:

"Leonard Thress, of 2618 Frankford Avenue, has learned how to live without eating. By physical experience he has proved not only that food is not a daily necessity of the human system, but that abstinence therefrom for protracted periods is beneficial. Indeed, it saved his life. He has just finished a fifty days' fast. When he began it he was on the brink of the grave and his physicians had abandoned hope. When he ended it he was in better health than he had enjoyed for years, although in the meantime he had lost seventy-six pounds, falling away from two hundred and nine to one hundred and thirty-three pounds.

"Thress, who is about fifty-seven years old, was attending the Grand Army Encampment at Buffalo in the fall of 1898, when he caught a violent cold, which settled in his bronchial tubes. It proved so stubborn that his general health became affected, and a year later dropsy developed. His condition grew steadily worse, and at Christmas time, 1899, it was such that he could neither walk nor lie prostrate, but was compelled to sit constantly in an armchair. His doctors exhausted their skill in the effort to bring relief, and eventually, in the early part of last January, they told him that their medicines refused to act, and that his death was a question of only a few days.

"Up to this time Thress had been subsisting on the meagre diet permitted to a man in his condition, but his stomach rebelled even at that. He had heard of the Dewey fasting cure and its boasted efficacy against all human ills, and, though he had little faith, death was already looming before him, and he knew that he could lose nothing by the experiment.

"He began to fast on January 11 by taking in the morning a portion of Henzel's preparation of salts in a glass of water and the juice of two oranges, and in the evening a hot lemonade. For twenty-five days he also drank a teaspoonful of a tonic consisting chiefly of iron, but the rest of the diet he continued until two weeks ago, when he discontinued the salts and orange juice and confined himself to a hot lemonade at morning and evening. This was his only sustenance until last Thursday.

"According to Thress's own recital, the effects of this course of treatment were amazing. He says that the natural craving for food was gone after the first day. Three days later he had regained so much strength that he was able to go upstairs to bed and enjoyed a good night's sleep. From that time on, although he steadily lost in weight, his vitality grew greater, and on January 22 he left the house and took a half-mile walk.

"Before three weeks of his fast had elapsed his dropsy had disappeared, and thereafter he took almost daily walks, increasing the distance with his strength. Some days he covered as many as five miles, and never less than two, even while he was growing thinner and thinner, as the accompanying table shows.

"For the first time since the beginning of his fast he became hungry last Thursday, March 1, and he felt that he should like some pigs' feet jelly. It is one of the prescriptions of the fasting cure that when hunger finally comes the patient shall eat whatever he craves, so Thress consumed two slices of the jelly and one piece of gluten bread, with butter. He says he enjoyed it and felt well afterward.

"He ate no more that day, but at noon yesterday he became hungry again, and this time his appetite was for something more substantial. He disposed of a dish of mashed potatoes, some red cabbage, another portion of pigs' feet jelly, apple sauce, and a cream puff for dessert. He even smoked a cigar after the meal, enjoyed it, and felt still better. He says he will eat no regular meals, but only when he becomes hungry.

"While he looks haggard and worn from the loss of flesh, Thress declares that all his ailments have left him and that he never felt healthier and heartier in his life."

"The following table shows how Thress grew stronger and walked miles while he was constantly losing weight from a fifty-days' fast:

		Weight.		
January	11	209		
"	12	207		
"	13	205		
"	14	202		
"	15	201		
"	16	200		
"	17	199		
"	18	196		
"	19	192		
"	20	190		
"	21	188		
"	22	186	Walked ½	mile.
"	23	180	" 2	miles.
"	24	177	" 2	"
"	25	172	" 3	"
"	26	167	" 3	"
"	27	165	" 3	"

"	28 162	"	2½	"
"	29 160	"	3	"
"	30 157			
"	31 155	"	3	"
February	1 154			
"	2 153			
"	3 152	"	3	"
"	4 151			
"	5 149	"	3	"
"	6 147	"	3	"
"	7 146	"	3	"
"	8 145			
"	9 145	"	4	"
"	10 145	"	4	"
"	11 145			
"	12 145	"	4	"
"	13 145			
"	14 145	"	3	"
"	15 144	"	2	"
"	16 142			
"	17 140			
"	18 140			
"	19 140			
"	20 138	"	2	"
"	21 137	"	4	"
"	22 135	Walked 3		miles.
"	23 135;	"	3	"
"	24 135			
"	25 135			
"	26 135			
"	27 133	"	2	"
"	28 133			

A. H. Potts, Editor of the *Chester County Times*, a man who has the largest faith in eating only to restore the wastes of the body, thus gives vent to his emotions after seeing the case by invitation of Mr. Ritter:

"On January 10 there sat in his home, at 2618 Frankford Avenue, Philadelphia, Mr. Leonard Thress, with dropsy, hopelessly given up to a speedy death by the many physicians he had vainly sought and paid well for relief. His weight was two hundred and nine pounds. His limbs were at the bursting point, and the water was close up to the top of his chest. He could not lie down nor even lay his head back without choking, and to walk across the room completely exhausted him. At that critical moment a friend of his heard of Miss Kuenzel's miraculous cure, and told him of it. He at once sent for Mr. Ritter, who thought that a cure was in his reach, and on January 11 Thress commenced a fast that has been absolute up to yesterday, the only things passing his lips being water, a little lemonade, and rarely the juice of an orange. Learning through the *Chester County Times* that we were interested in Dr. Dewey's discovery, he invited us to come and see the cases now under his care, and on Friday of last week we gladly availed ourselves of the opportunity to see the living proof of what we believed but had never seen. We were very cordially received at Mr. Ritter's home, and instead of meeting a pompous, egotistic, big man, as we might expect, we met a young gentleman of small stature, like ourselves, modest, retiring, and claiming no credit for his own part in these remarkable cures; but insisting that he is only observing the progress of cases, following in the line of truths discovered only by Dr. Dewey, giving such advice as he is enabled to do from his thorough knowledge of chemistry, anatomy, and hygiene. He took us to the house of Mr. Thress, and the startling impressions we received can never be effaced. We seemed to be in the presence of one who had arisen from the dead, and could not realize the truth of what we saw and heard from him and his estimable wife, who shows the happiness she feels in receiving her husband back to life. Impossible as it seems, yet on the previous day, as well as many other days, that man had walked three miles after six hours given to his business as a baker, which he now attends to personally. All traces of dropsy have disappeared, and his weight is now less than one hundred and thirty-five pounds, having lost this nearly seventy-five pounds of water through the natural channels at the rate of five or six pounds per day at times. His eyesight has grown younger and his hand is firm. He sleeps soundly several hours out of each twenty-four, and is almost a cured man, although the curative action is still going forward throughout his system, and his many friends are now awaiting the arrival of his normal healthy appetite, which in these cases does not arrive until the cure is entire, and then it comes in such a way as not to be mistaken. On Monday of this week we again visited him, taking a friend who has long suffered similarly to what he did, that she might see results for herself. We found him looking even better than on Friday, and it is very interesting to hear him tell his experience, which he will be glad to impart to those who are seeking after the truth, and interested in the cure of disease of themselves or their friends by this natural and without price (but priceless) means. We also visited two other of the five cases over which Mr. Ritter is at present keeping watch, and every one bore evidences of the great truth. No one should undertake the fast on their own responsibility, as certain conditions may arise requiring the eye of one who has made the matter a study, and no one should pass an opinion on the matter until they read Dr. Dewey's *New Gospel of Health*, wherein the reasons are made so plain that all can understand."

MR. LEONARD THRESS,
FIFTIETH DAY OF FAST.

Mr. Thress has regained his normal weight and has been in the best of health in the several months since the fast.[2]

The following case was deemed a miracle by all friends: Mrs. H. B., a woman of seventy-six, became exceedingly breathless, due, it was supposed, to defective heart action that had been chronic for many years. The final result was general dropsy. The eyelids had become so heavy that reading could be indulged only a short time because of their weight; the throat was also charged with water so as to make swallowing difficult. Beneath the eyes and jaws were pockets of water—in short, the skin of the entire body was distended, a condition that had deceived the friends as revealing only an increase of her natural stoutness. The real condition became known through a call to treat a bad cold.

What had authorized medical art to promise in such a case? Absolutely nothing, as she had become too old and weak to be subjected to the ordinary means for such a general condition. As for a fast for one so old, that was the last thing that would have been thought of: her age and debility would only have seemed to invite more daily food than she had been taking.

She was put on a fast, or rather the fast was continued, the cold having abolished her appetite. It went on until the fifteenth day, with increasing general strength and diminishing weight. The last days before hunger came she was able to go up a long flight of stairs without the aid of the railing and without marked loss of breath, the heart-murmur had nearly disappeared, and water by the gallon seemed to have been absorbed.

On the fifteenth day there was a desire for food, that was taken with relish through the enlarged throat without difficulty; the water pockets had become emptied, and the lids so thin and light as to reveal no fatigue in reading. Thence on one meal a day became the rule; and since there have been five years without any recurrence of the conditions—five years of remarkable general health and girl-time relish for her daily food.

How often has the cutting down of the daily food by the old and weak been condemned as too severe an ordeal to be safe! For this woman there have been these acquired years of nearly perfect health, and the end will be in the natural, easier death of old age.

The following is inserted as additional evidence of Nature's power over disease, and that brain-workers may go on with their labors with increasing power while waiting for natural hunger in cases in which hunger is possible:

Rev. C. H. Dalrymple, of Hampden, Mass., has just completed a fast, of which he says, February 5, 1900: "My fast continued thirty-nine and one-half days. My appetite came on me about 9 o'clock at night, and I thought I would wait until the next day; but two boiled eggs and some dry toast would not retire before my presence. I have never had such an assault upon my will power as that imagined egg and toast made on me. I was finally compelled to surrender. My tongue had been clearing up that day, and the next day I was hungry at noon. I have not missed a first-class appetite at noon since. My tongue has kept clear and my taste has remained sweet. I have had no chills nor fevers this winter, nor cold in any form. I have made no allowance for my sickness and have never worked harder. My flesh came back rapidly, and now I think I must weigh about fifteen pounds more than last summer. *I gained strength beyond all question about three weeks before my appetite returned. I would work all day long finally.* It was good to get well."

Mr. Ritter conducted over twenty cases, some being able to carry on their usual avocations. I give the most important ones: Mr. A. H., forty-five days; Miss B. H., forty-two days; Mrs. L., thirty-eight days; Mr. L. W., thirty-six days; Miss L. J., thirty-five days; Mrs. M., thirty-one days; Miss E. S., twenty-six days; Mr. G. R., twenty-five days; Mr. P. R., twenty-four days; and Miss E. Westing, forty-two days, who, on the fortieth day, was able to sing with unusual clearness and power, and ended her fast without losing a day from her duties as a teacher of music.[3]

Wonderful are these fasts? Not in the physiological sense. These fasts went on with only increasing comfort by day and more refreshing sleep at night. It is quite another thing to endure the fasts of acute sickness, for such they all are. That life is maintained for days and weeks, even months, under pain, discomfort—under all the torturing conditions of such diseases as pneumonia, typhoid fever, or inflammatory rheumatism, is far more a matter to wonder over.

I may well wonder that Nature is powerful enough to cure the sick at all even under the wisest aid; but with me the abiding wonder is that physicians do not see that acute sickness is a loss of all the natural conditions of digestion, with the wasting bodies the clearest evidence that food is neither digested nor assimilated. I wonder with only increasing impatience that the stomach is not understood as a machine that Nature wills shall not be run to tax her resources when life is in the throes of disease.

I had not been long engaged in observing the evolution of cure through Nature when I began to suspect strongly, as before intimated, that fasting is the true "medicine for the mind diseased." Not less evident than the cure of various ailings would be the emergence of the soul into higher life, and in some instances from the depth of despair. As the scope of my vision constantly enlarged through multiplying experiences, I began to see great hopes of the cure of the gravest of all diseases—insanity—through a rigid application of this method in Nature. I gave the matter so much thought and study that I wrote a monograph on the subject with the idea of publishing it, but gave it up to the idea of telling my impressions in "The No-breakfast Plan."

There are the same structural changes in the evolution of insanity as in that of catarrh. There is a morbid structural basis in minds diseased, the abnormal mentality or morality being merely symptoms of a physical disease. Of all human legacies, structural weakness of the mental or moral sense is the most unfortunate.

I shall say no more about the forms of mental disease than that there is distinctively both intellectual and moral insanity as a direct result of disease of the intellectual and moral centres. This will be more clearly seen when I recall the fact that moral insanity in its worse form—the suicidal—often exists with such intellectual clearness that there is the greatest ingenuity displayed in carrying out self-destruction. These mind and soul centres are often gravely diseased without impairment of muscle energy: the furious strength of the insane is an abiding fear with all.

It is clear that weakness of structure so soft as brain, a substance which is on the dividing-line between liquids and solids, must be of the gravest form from the first: grave because so fragile, grave because the sick centres cannot rest as the broken arm, the sick body: these centres, regardless how sick, must continue to serve, even in abnormal ways.

The possibility of insanity must always be a matter of the degree of the primary structural weakness and the energy and persistence of the operative forces; on these must depend the mere gentle, persistent illusion, or that fury of mania which transforms man, the "image of the Creator," into a wild beast. That insanity, no matter what its form or degree, is an evolution from an ancestral structural legacy, not essentially different from the structural conditions evolved from those of any other chronic disease, I cannot have the slightest doubt, any more than I can have for the structural means for the cure.

There is nothing that so illustrates the civilization, the benevolence of the age and of the nations as these palaces we call hospitals for the insane. Whatever there is that can add comfort to the body, or charm to the tastes, or new life to the soul has its culmination in these palaces of wood and stone, with one great exception: the structural condition of the diseased centres indicating rest, even as the ulcer, wound, or fracture, has no part in the methods of cure.

The feeding is all done not at the time of hunger, but at the time of day. All patients are expected to eat no less than three meals a day, regardless of any desire for food and whether the patient spends all his time in bed in mindless apathy, whether pacing his room with meaningless tread, whether active in light service in the building or in heavy labor without. When there is refusal to eat it seems to be taken for granted that suicide by starvation is the design, and the pumping of food into the stomach through the nose is the common resort. There seems to be no thought that there may be no hunger in such cases, and no apprehension of any danger from not eating; that in this they follow the instincts of brutes. Would the desire for food not come and with a saner condition of mind if they were permitted their own ways of eating?

A physically strong woman, whom I knew well, was sent to a hospital for the insane in a generally bad state of mind, with destructive propensities marked. With no desire for food, and certainly with no mind to realize the need to eat without hunger, she naturally refused to eat. But for a time her meals were forced down her throat, a proceeding that taxed the strength of several strong arms.

Why were the meals not omitted long enough to cause such a reduction of strength as to make feeding less expensive in the outlay of others' muscle? The persistent refusal to eat resulted in a cessation of all efforts to enforce food; left to the gentler hands of Nature for a time, the mental hurricane subsided in great degree on the return of hunger, and long before there was an appreciable loss of weight or strength. In a few months this woman was able to return to her home, and with restored mind to tell me of the violent feedings she had endured.

Now let us look again to the structural conditions involved in diseases of the mind. There are those soft, pulpy centres from which emanate the highest powers of life: power to think, to admire, to rejoice, or to suffer; and we know how digestive power varies along the scale between ecstacy and despair. In mental disease there is the same abnormal structural change as in other local diseases; but for these sick mind-centres there is no rest. There must be still thinking and feeling, no matter how chaotic, to tax them, and there is no cheer to electrify the stomach into easy display of power. We may well marvel that powers so wonderful as the power to think, love, admire, see, hear, and feel are located in structures so fragile as the brain; and we may well marvel at the provision of the turret of flinty hardness to protect it from violence.

Now we are to consider these centres of energy as abnormally weak in all their structures at birth in those who become insane: these are the luckless legacies from the fathers and the mothers, and for how far back in the ancestral line we do not know. We are to consider that there is the same abnormal condition of the cerebral bloodvessels and of the softer intervascular structures as in other local diseases; and when you recall the fact that everything that worries, that adds discomfort to either mind or muscles, is a force that tends to develop weakness and disease, you will see how it applies in the evolution of insanity.

Shall these fragile centres be permitted to rest when overwork has made them sick, or is there any other rational means for their recovery? Shall they not be permitted to rest when abundantly able to keep physically nourished in a way that does not cause even the slightest shade of discomfort?

Again, let it be borne in mind that recovery from acute disease is attended with a revival of strength in every power that makes life worth living, and that every person not acutely sick who has fasted under my care or who has cut down the waste of brain power by less daily food has found the same revival of power. To this there have been no exceptions.

What do we fear in sickness? Is it disease or the wasting pounds? Since they will disappear when Nature would have the food-gate closed, since they reappear when there is the highest possible reach of mere relish, and when all the other senses have become more acute, and also when existence has become almost ecstatic, why ever oppress the weak or sick centres when Nature wills a rest?

The literature on the disease of the mind has become so massive in mere bulk, in its physiological refinements, that it would require time with a long reach into eternity to go through it; but it has not come to my knowledge that it contains any reference to the brain as a self-nourishing, self-charging dynamo; that therefore the stomach is only a machine whose use can well be omitted for long periods when these centres of moral and intellectual energy have become worried into disease, with rest the only means, the only need for all the recovery possible.

"Oh, you giants of the medical profession!" You who have been elected to preside over these great homes of the mentally wrecked because of your eminence in character, ability, experience, and professional attainments, do you deny the soundness of the physiology involved in this method of reaching health through Nature? Then let me array against you Alexander Haig, M. A., M. D. Oxon., F. R. C. P., Physician to the Metropolitan Hospital, and the Royal Hospital, and for Children and Women; late Casualty Physician to St. Bartholomew's Hospital. I quote from his exhaustive work, *Uric Acid in the Causation of Disease*:

"And now I come to the causes which led me to take too much albumen and to suffer severely; in *Fads of an Old Physician*, Dr. Keith refers to another work on diet, by Dr. Dewey, of Meadville, Pa., *The True Science of Living*, and the chief point in this book is that temporary, complete starvation till there is once more a healthy appetite is the best cure for a host of dyspepsia, debilities, depression, mental and bodily, and numerous other troubles, and that for similar less severe disturbances of nutrition the great remedy is to leave out the breakfast, so as to give the stomach a long rest of sixteen hours or more, with the object of allowing it to recuperate and accumulate secretions after the last meal of the previous day.

"It seems from internal evidence in Dr. Dewey's book, a copy of which I owe to Dr. Keith, that his plans have been completely successful in a large number of cases, *and it seems to me that his logic is unanswerable,* and that in his main contentions he is perfectly right.

"Having arrived at this conclusion, I proceeded forthwith to put the matter to the test of experience by placing myself on two meals a day—that is, I left out my breakfast—and the result was I ate such a good lunch at 1 P. M. that it was impossible to take anything more till dinner-time, 7.30 or 8 P. M.; so that I reduced myself at once from four meals a day to two. The result was exactly what Dr. Dewey describes. I felt extremely bright and well in the morning, and capable of very good work, both mental and bodily. At 1 P. M. I had keen hunger, even for dry bread; such hunger as I had not experienced for years. After lunch (breakfast) I felt a little bit dull and occasionally sleepy, and the mental work for the first hour or two after it was not as good as usual. About 5 P. M. I was very thirsty and had to have a drink of water, but there was not the least desire for food until several hours later; though by 7.30 or 8 P. M. I was able to manage another fairly good meal; and thus my meals automatically, so to speak, reduced themselves to two."

I also quote from his work on *Diet and Food,* page 10:

"It is also possible, by introducing more food than can possibly be digested, to overpower digestion so that nothing is digested and absorbed, and starvation results, a fact that has been brought to the front in the most interesting manner in the writings of Dr. Dewey."

And who is Dr. Keith? You know that he is one of the youngest physicians in all Scotland, even if he does possess eighty years that are no burden to him. I quote him from his *Fads of an Old Physician:*

"Dr. Dewey's grand means of cure now is abstinence for the time from all food, and this he carries out to a degree which must astonish most physicians of the present day, as well as their patients. During times of sickness, when there is no desire for food, he gives none till the desire comes, and then only if the state of the tongue and general condition show that the power of digestion has returned. This may be in a few days, or in severe cases, as of rheumatic fever, it may not be for forty days or even longer. He points out very forcibly that we have all a store of material laid up in the body which supplies what is required for keeping necessary functions of the system going, while no food can be usefully taken in the stomach. I had mentioned this provision in my *Plea*, and had stated that so long as it lasts it is sufficient to preserve life. I also suggested that it might be found that the waste of the body was less when this internal supply was alone trusted to, than when it was supplemented by food from without which the organs of nutrition were not in a condition to utilize. This, to my mind, Dr. Dewey has proved to be the fact, and no one can read his case without being convinced that it is so. He gives a most interesting table from Dr. Yeo, showing what textures of the body waste most rapidly in disease. Fat is at one end of the scale, and at the other the brain, which does not waste till all the other textures and organs are depleted to the utmost.

"In cases of slighter disease where the patient is able to be about or to carry on his business, but with discomfort, the same abstinence from all food is recommended. It is usually found that work can be done more easily, and that strength actually increases, although the starving may have to be kept up for several days. But the great *coup* in Dr. Dewey's practice is, that to improve or to preserve health he advises all to give up breakfast, and to fast till the mid-day meal. In this he has had a very large number of followers, very much to their advantage. It may be that the omission of breakfast is more needed and has greater effect in America than it would have on this side of the Atlantic. In America the meal is generally a very full one, made up in a large measure of a variety of hot cakes, also flesh food and tea or coffee. The other two meals of the day are full, 'square' meals likewise. I have seen much overfeeding in this country, but never to such a degree, and so generally, as I have seen in America and on American steamers. In one of the latter the cooking was the worst I ever met with, but the hard meat was swallowed all the same, and the consequences must have been grievous."

Are you still without any questioning of your authorized, established methods of treating the mentally sick? Then let me quote against you another man across the ocean, whose ability, learning, and professional attainments are of the highest order. I quote from *Air, Food, and Exercise*, by A. Rabagliati, M. A., M. D., F. R. C. S., Edin., a man with whom patient, exhaustive investigation is only a recreation:

"It has been shown by physiologists that certain tissues are absorbed and used before others. Dr. Dewey, of Pennsylvania, with whose views I am glad to find myself in general accord, and who seems to have made the same attempt as the writer to view the facts of medical practice from an independent—and may I say, original?—standpoint, quotes a table of great significance from Dr. Yeo. Besides quoting it in the text of his book, *The True Science of Living*, Dr. Dewey places it in capital letters in the frontispiece of his book. He calls it Nature's Bill of Fare for the Sick; and he shows that in illness, when we are using up the materials accumulated in our bodies, we may use as much as 99 per cent. of our fat (practically all of it), that of muscle we may use as much as 30 per cent., that the spleen may waste to the extent of 63 per cent., the liver as much as 56 per cent., and the blood itself be absorbed to the extent of 17 per cent. of its total amount. But even when wasting to this extent has occurred the curious and significant fact is emphasized that the *brain and nerve-centres may not have wasted at all*. The controlling nervous system thus does not lose its powers till the very last. Generally, however, the wasting process does not require to be carried to the very last, the chronic inflammatory deposit (and in rare cases even a cancerous infiltration) being absorbed and got rid of before this point is reached.

"As most, if not all, of the chronic diseases depend upon the deposition of waste, unassimilated materials in various situations; or, in other words, depend upon a blocking of the local circulation in this way, a little wholesome starvation is generally of vast benefit by inducing the economy to use up some of its waste stuff. Nature herself points the way to us in this matter, because when things have gone as far as she can bear, and when, were things to go on in the same way, death must ensue, she generally throws the patient into bed with a digestive system entirely disorganized, taking away all appetite for food and all power of assimilation for the time being. We may, in such circumstances, do much harm by efforts too persistently made to feed our patients; but generally they refuse all sustenance for some time. After a while (Dr. Dewey does not seem to be afraid if his patients refuse all food even for as long on some occasions as thirty days continuously, or even longer) they right themselves, the tongue cleans, appetite returns, the power of assimilation is reëstablished, and recovery takes place. It strikes me as somewhat curious (and yet, if we both look at the facts of life candidly and impartially, perhaps it is not curious) that observers so wide apart, and in circumstances so very different as the conditions of human life must be in Yorkshire from what they are in Pennsylvania, should come to conclusions so practically similar as Dr. Dewey and the writer have reached."

Gentlemen, masters in the medical profession, to what good end are you pumping food into human stomach, where there is no hunger and no mind left to know the need? Is it to maintain that strength which costs you so much muscle at every feeding. Or is it that it would be a danger to lose a few pounds of body while Nature gets ready to ask for food in the gentlest and most persuasive way? Whatever there is in appeal to the best in any human life to uplift it from the deepest depths, you have at the readiest command. You seem amply equipped to reach everything but those sick, afflicted, oppressed brain-centres. You treat everything but these, but to these you are worse than the Egyptian task-masters in that you force needless labor where rest alone is the need. It is not bricks without straw, but labor with exhausted power; and for all your efforts you simply maintain weight at a tremendous cost to the energy of cure. In no class of patients is rest for the brain more indicated than in yours; in none are the means so at command and the results for good so promising. With your patients the importance of time for business or social use is no more a concern; the abnormal is all due to disease.

Let us consider those rooms of bedlam you call the "excitable wards." They who enter leave all hope (of the friends) behind. Is there special need in these regions of despair and mental chaos that the mere pounds and strength shall be kept up? What will be lost by protracted fasts? Nothing in the kitchen. As for the brain and those sick centres, they will feed themselves until the last heart-beat sends the last available nourishment to the remotest cell. Will the functions of the brain grow more abnormal by a suspension of digestive drafts upon it? Does rest to anything that is tired tend to the abnormal?

Again I ask, What will be lost by protracted fasts in such cases? Nothing but weight, of which the fat will be by far the larger part. Would there be worry about starvation? With most of the cases there is not mind enough to worry over anything from the standpoint of reason. The very fact of the absence of the sense of the importance of daily food would render fasts in the highest degree practical and successful.

The fasts could be instituted with the certainty of a calmer condition of mind as soon as the digestive tract would cease to call upon the brain for power, and with the probability that a surprising degree of improvement would be manifest in all, and long before the available body-food for the brain would be exhausted.

Gentlemen, you have treated acute sickness in all its forms, and you have had many cases in which, because of irritable stomachs, neither food nor medicine could be given. Day after day you have seen the wasting of the bodies, and you have also seen mental aberration or stupor lessen day by day as the disease lessened its grasp upon the brain-centres, and finally when the point of natural hunger was reached, you never found the lost pounds a matter of physical discomfort or mental abnormality or weakness; rather you have always found at this point a mental condition in every way the most highly satisfactory. I never saw brighter eyes, a happier expression on every line, than revealed by a woman after a fast of forty-four days, in which acute disease had reduced the weight forty pounds.

All overweight not due to dropsy or other disease is due to eating more food than the waste demands. As an abnormal condition overweight has received a great deal of attention in the way of misguided effort to both prevention and cure. These efforts are such conspicuous failures that even the patent medicine man has not found his "anti-fat nostrums" the happy means to fortune. There have been all kinds of limits built around bills of fare, but sooner or later Nature revolts and they are given up.

The reason that certain people take on weight easily and become "stout," is because of constitutional tendency, good digestion, and excess of food. As a general fact, the overweights are "large feeders," and they not only look well but feel well, for they have much less stomach trouble than the average mortal, and in cheerful endowment of soul they rank the highest among all the people.

In spite of my philosophy, I, who am one of the leanest of the kind, look upon the stoutness of those in the early prime of life with something of both envy and admiration; they seem so ideally conditioned to enjoy the best of all things on earth. But it is quite a serious matter when the muscles and brain have to deal with pounds in excess by the score, even as if the victim were doomed to wear clothes padded with so many pounds of shot.

Why some people take on fat easily even with the smallest of meals, why some of the largest eaters are of the leanest, are matters to talk about but not to know about. For my purpose it is sufficient that I assert that overweight can be prevented by an habitual limitation of the daily food to the daily need; that it can be cut down to any desired degree by stopping the supply, a method that is not attended with any violence to the constitution, nor even to comfort or power. This plan has the great advantage of adding to the curative energy of disease as well; and more than this, there is a change attending the loss that seems at first phenomenal, as involving a physiological contradiction—there is an actual increase in muscle-weight as the bloat and fat weight go down.

How is this, you ask? Here is the explanation: As the fat weight increases by surplus food, so decrease the disposition and ability for general exercise. As it declines, so do muscle and all the other energies increase, and the use of muscle within physiological limit tends to restore the normal weight and strength.

There are no overweights who would not receive the greatest benefit by a fast that would diminish the pounds to that of the ripest maturity of life, a fast that would be determined by the time required to reach the desired number of pounds. As a means this method is available to all, and practical where due physiological light will enable it to be carried out with no starving concern to disable vital power.

As a general fact, the No-breakfast Plan has been attended by a highly satisfactory reduction of surplus pounds; where there has been a failure it has been due to such an increase of digestive power as really to add to both an increase of the average amount of daily food and of power to digest it. For instance, one of my fellow citizens, weighing not less than three hundred and thirty pounds some years ago, gave up his morning meals. This was attended with entire relief from frequent bilious spells; but the average of daily food was increased and the business of a barber did not add anything to muscle development. Finally from mere excess of weight he became a prisoner to his house and yard, unable to walk a square without the greatest difficulty; and yet there were two enormous meals put into a stomach daily that did not complain, and the weight increased until the three hundred and seventy-five pound notch was nearly reached. He heard about the Rathbun fast, and I was able to persuade him to come down to one light meal daily, and day after day bonds were loosened. After a year there have been nearly seventy-five pounds lost, and there is ability to labor and to walk several miles daily.

Very many thin persons have gained as high as forty pounds by reason of the larger degree of muscle exercise. Since last writing, this word has come from Miss K., who one year ago was at the asylum eating several meals a day in bed with suicidal intent. She left that bed with a weight of one hundred and forty pounds, and, as I have mentioned before, lost twenty pounds of it by her fast. My last news is from a letter written the day after a twenty-five-mile ride among the mountains with a soul as free and joyous as there are freedom and joy with the birds whose songs greeted her rapt ears from every treetop. She writes of a gain of twenty-four pounds since the fast, and states that the glasses she has worn for thirteen years are wanted no longer!

I feel that I need not multiply words as to the ability and utility of bringing all overweight down to the physiological normal and of keeping it there. I could fill hundreds of pages with the joyous testimonies of those who have been relieved of many surplus pounds, with numerous accompanying ailings; they all tell the same story, and I will only add this, that there is no physiological excuse for any mortal to carry around weight that disables.

Not very many months ago ex-Governor Flower, of New York, a statesman of national fame, a man of largest public spirit, a most valuable citizen, and Colonel Robert Ingersoll, an orator of world-wide fame and of great nobility of soul, dropped as beeves beneath the stroke of an ax because of a fracture of brittle bloodvessels. In both of these cases not many less pounds than a hundred had needlessly accumulated.

Could I have had the Colonel's ear when I last saw him as a listener to almost matchless oratory, whose rotundity of belt was to be measured by the yard, I would have addressed him as follows: "My dear Colonel, when I last saw you you were just filled out enough to be the joy of your tailor, and as a picture of health in form and looks you were ideal. You were then eating the meals of a woodchopper; and merely because food tastes good and does not seem to hurt you, you have been doing the same during the nearly score and a half of years since I have seen you. You have been eating more food every day in proportion to general muscle exercise than the hardest toiler does in a week, and your vast bulk evidences against you."

After explaining to him the structural possibilities of apoplexy as a legacy, as I have to you in the cases of insanity, I would continue: "Now by virtue of a possible ancestral weakness of your brain arteries this may happen: the arterial walls, because of habitual food in excess, may undergo a fatty, limy degeneration that will make a rupture possible, with death or paralysis of one-half or more of the body as the direct result; or the small arteries may have their walls so thickened as not to permit enough blood to circulate in order duly to nourish parts of the brain they supply; hence softening of the structure and more or less imbecility.

"The history of all overweights is that of a decline of muscle energy, and very generally of the amount of muscle activity as the pounds and years increase; but no cut in the amount of daily food so long as it can be taken with relish and disposed of without any special protesting from the stomach. This is the history of by far the largest majority of those sudden deaths due to cerebral hemorrhage, and also the history of most of the cases of imbecility with the overweights.

"Now, Colonel, you should make a radical parting with those surplus pounds by a fast that may extend into months, or take one of the lightest of meals once a day. Follow this out rigidly until you have lost a hundred pounds, and then by as much will you be not only free from disease, but free also from the danger of disease."

My experience with cases of epilepsy, or "fits," is confined to a half dozen cases, in which permanent relief seems to be assured. There is an acquired structural abnormality behind the spasms, acquired from surplus food, with a cure to be reached ultimately in most cases along these physiological lines.

I shall not take time in telling the evils of alcoholics. It would not be more enlightening were I to spend hours in telling of wrecked lives, of wrecked homes, of prisons filled with their victims, of the immense loss to states and nations from the loss to sufferers and the loss they inflict. Alcoholism has no sense for frowning, ominous statistics, for it is a disease to be rationally treated, a disease to be rationally avoided.

In the light of later science the word "stimulants" has become a misnomer as applied to alcoholics; the term, no doubt, came into use from the fact that under their use there is more endurance to both physical and mental ills, an endurance or indifference ascribed to stimulation.

If power is stimulated by their use, then there should be a rise in temperature whereby severe cold is better endured; but this is not the fact any more than that temperature is lowered whereby extreme heat is endured; in either case the endurance is due to benumbed brain-centres. The alcoholic simply lessens the power to suffer mentally or physically; hence in degree it is an anæsthetic, and as such it also affects the moral sense and lessens the power of reason and judgment. They are habitually taken for no other reason than for the temporary relief they give to some ill of life.

It seems the very depths of total depravity when there is no bread for the hungry family, that the price of a loaf will rather be spent for a drink; but it is not so much moral depravity as depravity of brain-substance. The lethal drink is taken because without it there is more acute suffering than from the want of a loaf of bread by the entire family. In my practice an ordinarily sober father would always get drunk and stay drunk while any member of his family was sick, and for the sole reason that he could not endure the worry of apprehension. This was not so much depravity as an acute sense of the suffering and danger involved, a painful rousing of the best instincts of the soul, those instincts that raise man above the brute and make him the noblest work of the divine hand. That is not a bad man at heart who has such a sense of affection for his wife or child when they seem dangerously sick that he must have artificial aid to endurance; and if you shall detect the alcoholic odor in his breath at the funeral you may know that there is heart agony under repression.

The fact that alcoholics are anæsthetics, and not stimulants, has become known to a few of the scientists in the medical profession; but it can scarcely be said to have become known to the profession generally. That the habitual drinker partakes for any other reason than to drown his woes that will not stay drowned, and that the drowning is not stimulation, do not need argument.

The alcoholic in proportion to its strength is mental chaos and paralysis to power, and it has not the virtue to contain an atom that can be converted into a living atom. In not the least sense is it a tissue-builder, and its use by the medical profession is without the shadow of a reason, and is all the more reprehensible in cases of shock.

Let us see: shock in degree is brain paralysis; alcoholics in degree are brain paralyzers; shock is simply a state of exhaustion with rest the supreme need. All the rousement that is necessary and that can avail will be called into action by the need of oxygen. There are cases of disease in which breathing goes on hour after hour, when the soul seems to have departed and with it every life sense. The patient has become dead beyond reviving, and yet breathes hour after hour. Now can one for one moment think that an alcoholic can add to the power of the respiratory centres of the brain to respond to the calls for oxygen and so prolong life? Shock in its gravest degree is to be considered the extreme of the tired-out condition, with rest the only restorative means; and rest may be permitted with the certainty that for mere breathing purposes alcoholics are dangerous in proportion to the gravity of the shock.

In health the alcoholic only adds discomfort, because there are no complaints to soothe; hence it is the duty of every mother so to train her sons in health-habits that those first drinks will be discouraging because they bring no cheer of contrast, but rather sensations that are not suggestive of a better physical condition.

Alcoholics have a corroding effect upon the mucous membrane of the stomach, a congestive effect by which the glands are subjected to starving pressure; hence their use always disables the mere mechanics and the chemistry involved in digestion, and so prolongs disease, and this applies to all medicines that corrode. This corroding power of the alcoholics upon the walls of the stomach and its paralyzing effect upon the brain-centres, with the additional fact that there is nothing in it that adds force to any life power or that can be converted into living atoms, should make its use in the stomach of the sick a crime scarcely to be excused by ignorance.

The evolution of the drunkard is a process of culture, and involves something of a constitutional tendency as in other diseases. I conceive that there is an alcoholic temperament, or a temperament in which the inability to bear with patience the various mental and physical woes of life is marked even from childhood. Indigestion and every cause that lowers vital power only add to the importance of such a nervous system.

The first step in the evolution of the drunkard is the first untimely meal drawn from the breast of the mother. By irregular nursings and the nursings merely to stop crying the nervous system is continually overtaxed. There are the untimely meals to prevent gluttony; there are the between-meal lunches to incite nervousness, irritability, a feeling of unrest that nothing seems to satisfy.

This goes on year after year until the time comes when that first drink has power to soothe many discordant voices, and the die is cast. Other drinks follow, with each to lessen the power of the dynamo and to disable the machine. At first, drink is indulged not without a sense of wrongdoing, but with that feeling of power in reserve to keep within the limits of safety.

The gradual corrosion of the stomach adding to the labors of the brain in the matter of food mass decomposition as well as digestion marks the decline of power to abstain and the degradation of every sense that makes life worth living. Now add to the corrosion of the membrane and the paralysis of the brain-centres from alcoholics the other inciting causes in the culture of disease, and you have the evolution of the drunkard.

How is he to be cured? Only through a fast that shall let that diseased stomach become new from regeneration, that will let the brain accumulate rest in reserve. For a time you will need to have him under bonds, for his will power is abolished. Put him where there will be deaf ears to the cries of morbid nature, for there is to be a conflict at first; but long before hunger will come the storm will subside; and finally, when food will be really desired, there will be a new stomach and a new brain to which an alcoholic will be no temptation.

This is no figure of speech, because there is such a continual change of life and death going on in the soft tissues of the body that in a month or more of fasting it may be assumed that much of the tissues which is left has undergone reconstruction, and both brain and stomach act as if they are new when the time comes to restore the lost pounds.

The ways of the kitchen and dining-room are the ways of disease and death, ways whose ends are prisons, asylums, scaffolds, to a far larger extent than is dreamed of by the fathers and mothers of the land. A new crusade against intemperance, the intemperance of the dining-room, is the only one that will ever settle this so-called liquor question. The rum-seller will only pull down his sign through the starvation of his business.

With brains and stomachs kept in the highest order, the alcoholic has only the least power of the beguiling kind; it is rather a dose whose effects do not invite repetition. But for all who have the drink disease seemingly beyond hope a fast of a month, or two months if necessary, will cure any stomach or brain, no matter how pickled they are with alcoholic soaking, and with only the least disturbance in the habit breaking; even within a week the hardest of the fighting should be over when the fast is made absolute.

I have now to consider briefly a most distressing disease, one that perhaps was never cured by the power of doses, and that most happily illustrates the structural changes in the cure of disease.

Asthmatic distress is caused by congestion of the terminals of the bronchial tubes, by which entrance of air into the cells is made difficult, even in some cases to the point of suffocation. This condition as a disease may be called bronchial catarrh, as in most cases there is such a condition of the larger tubes as to cause the habitual raising of a discharge. As to the disease itself, you have only to recall what has been said about nasal catarrh in order to understand its origin and development. It would be as trivial a disease were it not for the fact that those smaller and ultimate tubes, because of flabby walls and weak vessels, become congested, with resulting narrowing of the air-ways of life.

For this most distressing disease local treatments are as futile and void of intelligence as the physiology and anatomy involved in cause and cure of other local diseases. Is it not a great thing that those too narrow ways of life may be reached through a fast which shall so charge the brain with power that the flabby walls will be condensed; that most cases of asthma may be cured, with marked relief for every case? This is as certain as a result, as that rest restores strength. With the toning of the brain through rest, a catarrh of the bronchial tubes is certainly curable in most cases. With a large opportunity to know I am able to say this with intense conviction.

Only a few months ago, just before the break of day, a freight train took a side track; in a few moments, with nearly a mile-a-minute speed, a limited passenger train took the same track, and in the time of a second five men were hurled into eternity. Why? How? The conductor and his brakeman were in such heavy sleep when the switch was opened that they were not awakened to close it.

Why? How? There was the torpor of indigestion holding the tired brains of those two men in its fatal grasp; their stomachs were full of food when they were already tired out by their long trip that was nearly at its close, and for them those untimely meals were the last.

Of all men who ought to work with empty stomachs for the sake of the best possible reach of the memory it is the railroad engineer and conductor; so also every man who is in any way responsible for the safety of the trains. If we had the history of all the derailments, collisions, of cars with human freight converted into funeral pyres, a frightful percentage of them could be traced to where "some one had blundered" because of the torpor from handling meals when the brain was compelled to higher services. Digestive, indigestive torpor is also torpor of the sense of *responsibility*.

In the city where I live is the point between two divisions of the Erie Railroad, each somewhat more than a hundred miles long. Before I began the agitation of the No-breakfast Plan all trainmen felt that filling their stomachs was the last duty before entering upon their taxing trips, and tired wives would have to get up at all times of the night to prepare general meals. In this city a mighty revolution for the good of wives, for the good of men themselves, and for the safety of the trains and the hapless passengers has been going on for some years.

In former times when these men came home from their rounds generally tired out, and with a feeling that in proportion to the sense of exhaustion was the need to eat, general meals had to be prepared at any time of night. All this is changed in a large measure. Trainmen have been finding out that the less food in their stomachs they take into bed with them and on to their trains, the better it is for them in every way.

More and more they are getting into the way of having a general meal when they can eat it with leisure and leisurely digest it; and I predict that a time will come when all who are in any way responsible for the running of trains will have to know how to take care of their stomachs, in order that they shall attain and maintain the highest efficiency for services where human lives so much depend on the best there is in memory, reason, and judgment. This will be a part of their preparatory education.

The "block system" has wonderfully added to the safety of the trains, but there should be a block system added to the stomachs of the dispatchers and all whose duties are so grave as the handling of human freight. There is no division so long that it cannot be doubled with less fatigue and better mental condition if the stomach be not on duty at the same time. In this I speak with the authority that comes from the study of the experiences of trainmen during many years: with one accord they speak of their trips as taken with clearer heads and stronger muscles than when large meals were thought a necessity while on duty.

With an empty stomach it takes a very long time to get into such torpor—drowsiness—as compels the after-dinner sleep. That engineer who once told me of such sleepiness as made him nod while on duty was not suffering from either lack of sleep or overwork of his body: it was simply a case of the torpor of indigestion, and this was when there was no block system to lessen the danger of such services.

There is a great deal of imperfection in what man does for man that comes from the indifference arising from the torpor of untimely food, and far more than there is any conception in what man does against man from the destruction of power in this way.

There is now one of the Erie conductors who five years ago was losing at least half of his time from asthma; there is another who was equally disabled from sudden head symptoms that would immediately disable. These men have lost no trips since they began to run their stomachs with the same care as their trains. And there is an engineer whose trips to the physician and to the drug-store for many years were as frequent as those to his engine. There has since been a half dozen years of wiser care of his stomach, and his wife says that the change for the better in his disposition is beyond description. These men have rendered far more service, and who cannot see that these services have been of far higher character for the company, and that they have been infinitely better husbands, fathers, and citizens?

The following case will interest trainmen: D. S., a brakeman, reached the burden of two hundred and forty-six pounds, with resulting breathlessness and other ailings that taxed all his resources to perform his duties. He was induced to cut down his daily food as the only means for relief, and to add to his strength. It took him a long time to master the fact that his strength was not kept up by food, but the gradual loss of weight with the general improvement made this more and more evident. He finally reached a time when he was able to make his round trip of one hundred and ninety-six miles without a morsel of food the while, and with much less fatigue than when there was a midnight meal from a lunch-pail. Within a year the weight has gone down to one hundred and eighty-eight pounds. To my professional eye there is beauty in the bright eyes, in the condensed, smooth face, in the body enfolded with clothes that flap in the breeze like the sails of a ship. No accident will happen to precious human freight through his brain kept free from digestive torpor while on duty.

Ever since my book has been out I have been in more or less trouble with cases that badly needed my personal care, and not few in which death was inevitable. For instance, there is a woman in Illinois who has been ailing for years, and in spite of the No-breakfast Plan has had to take to her bed with acute aversion to food. Medical art had utterly failed before she changed her dietary methods.

Her dietary views are known, and so she is held in severe censure because the sick stomach is not compelled to a futile service; and though I am informed of an enlargement in the region of the bowels that has been perceptible and tender for years, her death will be considered suicidal from *starvation*.

A Warrensburg, Ill., editor began his fast by throwing up his food and continued it to the end; yet because he had talked about a fast it was supposed to be a case of suicide of the stupid kind; and though the post-mortem revealed a diseased gall-bladder, the doctors who made it did nothing to lessen the suicidal impression, and the death from "starvation" appeared under large headlines in the public prints.

When men as learned, able, and eminent as Dr. Shrady, of New York, go into print to inform the public that people may starve to death in ten days, and when such men as Prof. Wood, of the University of Pennsylvania, do not see any starvation in the wasting pounds of acute disease, the care of acute sickness as Nature would have it is a grave matter for the physician.

In five fatal cases under my care in which there was no possibility of feeding, there was such agitation over the question of starvation as would have subjected me to violence had my city been nearer the equator. In all these cases I was compelled to have a post-mortem to silence heathen raging. In one case in which a young man had died after weeks of inability to take food, even one of my medical brethren carried the conviction with him for years, and without seeking to inform himself, that there was a death from starvation. In this case there were spells of hunger in a fury, when meals would be taken, only to be soon thrown up, and he finally took to his bed to starve slowly to death. There was mind enough left to make a will, though the body had lost apparently more than half the normal weight; the post-mortem revealed a stomach seared, thickened, and not more than a third of the normal size.

The physiology of fasting in time of sickness is so entirely new to the medical world that every death that occurs with those who practise it is certain to be attributed to starving.

Early in this year (1900) a woman of seventy, in high circles, died from an obscure stomach trouble. For thirty-eight days there averaged nearly a half-dozen spells of vomiting; and yet it was generally believed that it was clearly a case of death from starvation, believed by those whose power to receive impressions is far stronger than their power to consider.

Fasting, because it is Nature's plan, will win the victory in all cases in which victory is possible; and yet wherever it is adopted, to become known about, there will be the same confusion of tongues as would be were violent hands laid upon gods of wood and stone in heathen temples. "Starved to death" is the verdict.

Fasting during sickness, because of the vast utility and from the impetus arising from the cases in Philadelphia, is bound to spread as by contagion; but when death occurs, all friends involved will be charged as abettors of homicide. To be fair to the opposition, and to let all readers know what chances for public censure will be theirs, whenever they see fit to let their friends recover on Nature's plan or die natural deaths, the following case is given. I quote from the Philadelphia *Press* of May 7, 1900:

"In the death notices of April 26 appeared the name of Mrs. Hermina Meyer, fifty years of age, of 1233 North Howard Street. At the time this short and simple record of the passing away of an ordinary, obscure woman attracted no more attention than the hundred similar names that constituted the necrological annals of April 25. But there is a startling aftermath that at once gives significance to this brief record, and rude and bitter awakening to the followers of the so-called 'Starvation Cult,' that has gained a considerable acceptance in the northeast section of the city.

"Mrs. Meyer was a believer in the fasting treatment. She was apparently a victim of this strange and heretical therapeutical faith. Kensington is buzzing with gossip concerning the deplorable death of the unfortunate woman. C. F. Meyer, the husband of the victim, accepts the death of his wife as due to heart-failure, and apparently is not disposed to complain.

"Mr. Meyer talked freely with a *Press* reporter yesterday concerning the sickness and death of his wife. He said that Mrs. Meyer had been ill for about a year, her malady having been diagnosed as chronic rheumatism. She had been treated by the family physician for this disease, but without relief. In despair she turned to the fasting treatment.

"From time to time she had read of the remarkable cures claimed to have been effected by complete abstention from food. Through a friend she met and talked with the family of Leonard Thress, of 2618 Frankford Avenue, whose case is proclaimed as one of the most remarkable that had been successfully treated by the fasting system. Thress was widely advertised as a victim of dropsy, who, after a complete fast of more than a month, was restored to sound health.

"Mrs. Meyer believed, and sent for Henry Ritter, the chief advocate and adviser of the fasting cult in Philadelphia. His belief in the weird treatment of disease he has adopted is seemingly unshakable.

"Ritter has superintended many cases of starvation treatment, wherein, according to his own statements, the patients have totally abstained from actual food for periods of from four to six weeks. He claims that in every case the afflicted person has completely recovered health—with the single exception of Mrs. Meyer.

"In response to her request, Ritter called upon Mrs. Meyer. She at once began her fast. Nothing was allowed to pass her lips but a small quantity of tonicum and some physiological salts, dissolved in water. Of each of these she was permitted to take sparingly every day. It is claimed by Ritter, a fact well-known to physiologists, that there is no actual food in either of these thin condiments. They are simply stimulants. These liquids, according to Ritter, are the only things given to any of the patients whose cases he has supervised.

"For twenty-five days, so says Mr. Meyer, his wife fasted and improved. At the expiration of that time, he says, her health was very much improved. She was able to walk about her room, a thing she had not been able to do for many weeks. Then there was a sudden and violent change for the worse. The patient was seized with convulsive vomiting.

"For sixteen days she suffered the excruciating pains of these convulsions. But, under Ritter's advice, Mrs. Meyer continued her fast. Till the thirty-fifth day she tasted no food. The vomiting continued unabated. On the thirty-sixth day she felt a craving for food for the first time since her long fast began. She was given oatmeal porridge. But the vomiting continued unabated.

"She grew weaker and weaker. From one hundred and fifty pounds weight she was reduced to a gaunt skeleton. When, upon the resumption of a food diet, the vomiting did not cease, the family was alarmed. The family physician was sent for in dismay. But he could do nothing. Flesh-building foods were prescribed, but they accomplished nothing. The vomiting continued, and three weeks following the breaking of the fast Mrs. Meyer died.

"The death was put down to a depleted blood-supply, or heart-failure. Ritter claimed that this unexpected turn could not have been anticipated, as the fact that the patient was subject to heart disease was previously unknown.

"He had treated her for rheumatism, and the cure was apparently in sight when heart-failure carried the patient to her grave.

"These facts were detailed by Mr. Meyer. He added that Mr. Ritter was not a physician; that he charged no fees; that he did not claim to prescribe remedies, but only advised.

"So ends the case of Mrs. Hermina Meyers, first victim of the starvation cult."

The following is from the *Press* of May 8:

"The death of Mrs. Hermina Meyer, after undergoing the fasting treatment for thirty-five days, has not at all shaken the faith of the adviser responsible for the ordeal, Henry Ritter, who claims to have restored tireless persons to health. He affirmed that the ravages of chronic disease had progressed too far for his treatment to conquer them, and that his attendance was advised by the family physician.

"Against this comforting declaration, however, stands the fact that the certificate of death, signed by Dr. James Chestnut, Jr., gave as the cause prolonged abstinence from food; in other words, *starvation*. Dr. Chestnut also has stated that the case was taken out of his hands, and Ritter installed as medical adviser, by what was virtually a dismissal. Dr. Chestnut was summoned again when the condition of the woman became critical, after twenty-five days of fasting, but she became rapidly weaker with violent convulsions and vomiting, and was beyond medical aid.

"She had never been treated for cancer of the stomach, which Ritter says he thinks she may have had, although she had a valvular affection of the heart which had existed for some time. But the fact that the cause of her death was officially attested by the family physician as due to her long fast contradicts flatly the position taken by the self-constituted healer, who made the following statement last night:

"'I have seen all the members of Mrs. Meyer's family to-day, and they are entirely satisfied that my treatment was in no way responsible for her death. I was called in at their urgent request, as their own relatives were numbered among the cures to the credit of the fasting treatment, as well as Mr. Thress. I accept no money for my work; they knew it was a labor of love, and the family physician, Dr. Chestnut, agreed with them as to the advisability of this system which they had seen tested.

"'Mrs. Meyer improved rapidly for a time, her chronic rheumatism causing her less trouble than in years, after the first three weeks of fasting. She had been treated previously for catarrh of the stomach, and it is probable that a cancer afflicted her. I am using no new system. The method has been used with very notable success by Dr. Edward H. Dewey, of Meadville, whose reputation and standing are distinguished. This is the first case I have lost out of twelve patients who had been given up as hopeless by regular physicians. It is Nature's cure, nothing more; but it was applied too late in the case of Mrs. Meyer.'

"Dr. Chestnut would not allow himself to be quoted because of the rigid rules of medical ethics. It may be stated, however, in addition to what has been said, that he does not wish to be considered as having encouraged the experiment, and that the death certificate defined his view of the responsibility."

A verdict on the part of the doctor *without a post-mortem*.

Against the doctor is the following, from the daughter, Miss Kate Meyer. I quote from an article in the *North American* of May 8, 1900:

"Mrs. Hermina Meyer, devotee of an odd cult, that regards starvation as a sure cure for all bodily ills, fasted for nearly forty days because she was suffering from rheumatism.

"The rheumatism disappeared.

"But after twenty-five days of total abstinence from food she sickened. Violent nausea came to her. She died.

"Nevertheless, Miss Kate Meyer, daughter of the dead woman, says:

"'My mother did not die because she fasted. The fasting did her good. When she began it she had been ill with rheumatism for more than a year. She could hardly walk. Her left arm was powerless. She could not lift it from her side. After two weeks of fasting she was active. She could walk. The power came back to her arm. She suffered little pain. She looked well. Then came the attacks of nausea.

"'But Dr. Chestnut, who is our family physician, was attending mother all the time. He called once a week. He said himself that the fast cure seemed to be doing mother good. When she got nausea he did not lay it to her fasting. He said it was heart trouble. That's what mother died of. Dr. Chestnut said so.

"'Do you remember the case of Leonard Thress? He cured himself of dropsy by fasting. Mother heard of it. She was introduced to Mr. Thress. He told her that all he knew of the fast cure he had learned from Henry Ritter. Mother sent and asked Mr. Ritter about the cure. Then she began it. Mr. Ritter never charged mother for anything. Dr. Chestnut consented that mother should try the Ritter cure.'

"Mrs. Meyer was the wife of Charles F. Meyer, of 1233 North Howard Street. Meyer, like his daughter, has only friendliness for Ritter, and also favors the fast cure. Mrs. Meyer, past middle age, had been sorely tried by her ailment. For more than a year Dr. Chestnut attended her, but her condition did not improve. Prescription after prescription was tested, only to fail.

"'There is little hope for me,' said the woman to her daughter. 'I'm tired of taking medicines. They do me no good.'

"She became more melancholy as the days passed. She regarded her case as hopeless. Dr. Chestnut acknowledged defeat. He had only a change of climate—a long stay in Colorado—to recommend. A very domestic woman was Mrs. Meyer. She looked with horror upon a journey. She said she would remain at home and die.

"But one day last March there gathered at a banquet in the home of Leonard Thress about a dozen persons, very happy, very healthy (or believing themselves to be so), all members of the 'starvation cure' cult.

"Each had to tell the story of a long fast that brought a remarkable cure. Newspapers gave publicity to the dinner of the little band with the odd faith in fasting. Mrs. Meyer heard of it. Here was a chance—a gleam of hope! She came to know Leonard Thress, and, through him, Henry Ritter, the apostle of the fast cure. He told her of remarkable recoveries. She caught his enthusiasm.

"But, according to Mr. Meyer, the young man was careful first that the family physician should consent. He never hinted at compensation for his services; never got it. Aside from advising total abstinence from food, he supplied small quantities of tonicum and salts dissolved in water. These contained no food matter; they were merely stimulative.

"In two weeks hope was strong with Mrs. Meyer; with all the family. Certainly, she was improving. She could walk; her arm that had been stiff and painful moved with ease—hurt no more. She still suffered occasional twinges, and decided to continue her self-imposed starvation until every rheumatic germ in her body was eradicated.

"She regarded herself as almost cured, when, after twenty-five days, she was attacked with nausea. She was very ill. It lasted sixteen days. After the first few days of fasting all desire for food had vanished. But on the thirty-sixth day she was hungry.

"Oatmeal porridge was given her sparingly. The nausea, however, did not cease. She began to grow alarmingly emaciated. She had weighed one hundred and fifty pounds. Her weight had fallen to one hundred.

"The family physician prescribed light food, but her stomach repulsed it. She grew very weak.

"On April 26 she died. Dr. Chestnut unhesitatingly issued a death certificate, ascribing her death to heart-failure. He also suspected a cancer of the stomach, but was not sure.

"Mrs. Herman Reinhardt, a cousin of the deceased woman, is firmly convinced that fasting had nothing to do with her death.

"'For more than fifteen years Mrs. Meyer suffered from some acute stomach trouble,' Mrs. Reinhardt said yesterday, 'and it is my belief that it caused her death. Her general health had been greatly benefited by abstaining from all food, but the disorder from which she suffered most could not be cured. My husband fasted for twenty-five days and was completely cured of stomach trouble, and there were no ill effects in his case.'"

The impression of this death and of these fasts upon the minds of the medical profession was perhaps fairly summed up by the eminent Horatio C. Wood, M. D., LL. D., Clinical Professor of Nervous Diseases in the University of Pennsylvania. He disregarded the legal phase of the question, the question of the legality of a layman dealing out words of cheer and comfort in cases in which the medical profession had retired in total defeat. The question had been seriously raised as to whether Mr. Ritter had not committed a crime against the laws of Pennsylvania, and for what? For simply advising these people to stop all eating until there would come a natural desire for food!

Professor Wood thus gave utterance in the *Press* of May 10:

"'These people are falsifying,' he said, 'There have been liars, you know, and they are not all dead. I don't believe for an instant such stories as fasting totally for forty or fifty days and keeping up energy and activity. It is contrary to common sense as well as to all we know about the human body. I don't know the object of deception, but somebody must be making money out of it, or having a craving for notoriety. It is preposterous. I understand that one of these fasters walked ten miles a day, after doing altogether without nourishment for a month or so. If these persons did what they claim to have undergone, more than one death would have been charged against the treatment, you may be sure.

"'You will remember that the professional forty-day fasters, Tanner and Suci, were reduced to mere skin and bone, were almost helpless, carefully husbanded every bit of their vital energy, and took no exercise. They were *watched* and studied scientifically. And here is a woman, weighing only one hundred pounds when she started fasting, claims she began to eat after thirty-eight days of starvation, and had more energy and took more exercise than in years. It is all amazingly absurd, whatever the motive may be.'"

Tanner and Suci, "skin and bones?" Cowen weighed one hundred and seventy-five pounds when he began his forty-two day fast, and lost only thirty pounds. My case of acute rheumatism revealed a loss of only forty pounds after a forty-six days' fast; and the woman of fifty-seven who began eating on the forty-third day was so well padded with muscle and fat as not to reveal the slightest suggestion of starvation as she sat down to the first meal. "Skin and bones?" This is a matter for months, and not for days.

"Falsifiers, these fasters?" Science settles important questions by investigation, not by epithet.

As I write the closing pages of this book, the most taxing case of fasting that ever came under my care has ended in hunger, and I insert it that all may know what tribulations will be theirs if they have any part in letting their sick get well or die in that peace God and Nature clearly design for all.

A man of large mould came to me, unknown, unbidden, from a distant city on the seventeenth day of his fast. His appetite had been abolished by a severe throat and bronchial attack, both of which had been relieved before reaching me. Well posted in the theory of fasting, he came with the declared intention of fasting until hunger or death would come.

For two or three weeks he was able to be about the city with his nearly two hundred pounds of flesh; but there was an unknown, unknowable disease of the bowels and stomach in slow development. There were a dryness of the mouth and such aversion to food as to forbid all eating, and he was deaf to my suggestion that he should at least taste some of the liquid foods from time to time, to save me in the eyes of his friends from a verdict of homicide, were we to fail to win a victory. After more than fifty days without even a taste of food nausea and vomiting were added to his woes, and when his friends became aware of the many days without food no words I could utter saved me from the severest condemnation. The anxiety that involved the sick bed only depressed the patient, and when another physician had to be called to relieve the pressure the last hope with him nearly departed.

The adviser was a man of high character and of unusual general and professional acquirements. Behind him was the entire medical profession and all its literature: behind me were only Nature, many-voiced—and the patient. With us there was no lack of mutual respect, except in matters of faith and practice; but he no more tolerated my "crankiness," lunacy—perhaps imbecility—in withholding food from the sick than I his paganism in enforcing it. For the sake of the agony of friends my noble patient accepted one severe dose of medicine and one ration of predigested food.

The instant response of the digestive powers was, "We have stopped business down here for repairs: when we are ready we will let you know."

Next a ration of food was sent into the sick bowels, only to cause hours of pain. The enemy having been expelled with disaster from all points of attack, there simply had to be a waiting on Nature, and in one day after the last vomiting spell there was a natural call for food—and this on the *sixtieth day of the fast!*

Had this man died—such was his prominence—I should have been paraded as a criminal of the stupid kind in the entire press of America, except in the papers of my own city. For this man of sixty-five, who with marvellous faith in Nature patiently waited upon her time, there promises to be many years of the days of his youth restored to him. As for me, with authorized medicine driven from the field, I see only new life unfolding in him daily, and my reward is exceeding.

Men and brethren of the medical profession: This man read his favorite *Sun* during every one of those sixty long days, and not one day was there revealed a hint of mental loss in clearness of apprehension. He lived because he knew that starving to death was his remotest danger; he lived also because he was made to see evidences that a cure was evolving in many ways. There was at no time apprehension, except when he felt unable to resist his friends with a *No* in thunder tones when it was proposed to torture him with drugs and foods.

Brethren, are you going into print to denounce the physiology or the practicality of this old method in Nature, this new method in humanity, to the sick and afflicted? Not one of you can advance arguments that will convince those who reason.

To what good end are you now enforcing your *predigested* foods? Are they relished better than other foods? Can they be taken with less aversion in cases of nausea and vomiting? Do they really nourish the brain so as to add clearness and strength to the mind? Do they ever prevent the uncovering of bones that makes the ways of acute sickness? If food actually can be so digested out of the body as to be ready for instant absorption, we should be able to abolish our kitchens, and at once enter upon that golden age in which there would be no dyspepsia hydraheaded; no disease of any kind, not even drunkenness, and where death would be only as the last flicker of the burned-up candle.

In this case, as in all other cases, the desire for water was abolished before hunger became marked. In this connection I will suggest to the reader that thirst is a morbid condition to be avoided as far as possible; that water is its only need, and no mortal ever needs a drop for health's sake except when thirsty. Making water-tanks of human stomachs is without the shade of physiological reason, and the alleged results for good are not based on a shade of scientific evidence: these are based wholly in the minds of the credulous enthusiasts who prescribe them. Taking large quantities of water without thirst only entails added work upon the kidneys, and thus it becomes a factor in the development of Bright's disease and other forms where the tendency exists. The actual need of water is always made clear in every case; the need always disappears before hunger can become possible.

As to the use of water on the body, this physiology has to be taken into account. The skin is covered with scales that are constantly dropping off as they mature, each to uncover a bright, clean one. As the skin is not an absorbent membrane, and as old scales are constantly dropping off, the need of frequent baths is more a need to satisfy the personal sense of cleanliness than a physiological need. These scales should not be either soaked off or brushed off in a wholesale way; the oil in the skin is a protection against weather-changes, and is also a necessity to its functional integrity, and therefore should not be dissolved and washed off by soaps that are strongly alkaline.

The body itself is very sensitive to contact with water below the natural temperature of the skin. The plunge bath is specially depressing to every human energy, and should never be indulged by the debilitated. The daily bathings of nursing children are cruel and life-depressing. Their little bodies are always clean in the physiological sense when their clothes are kept clean; hence once a week ought to satisfy all mothers.

The question of how often to bathe must be considered along these physiological lines. They whose employments soil their clothes and bodies spend the least time in cleansing their bodies; and yet in no medical work that treats of diseases and their causes is there to be found a hint that any special disease has its origin in uncleansed skin as a chronic condition. That will be a small-minded reader who draws conclusions from these statements that the author is not highly in favor of having bodies and clothes kept so habitually clean as not to be an offence to the finest fibred olfactory nerve at close range. In the use, then, of water on the body be physiologically sensible, and not the slaves of the bath-tub or "medicated" waters.

Lay readers, I draw my message to a close. I have addressed it to you because your minds are open and free. Draw near and listen while I talk rather than write. Let me look into your eyes, see the play on all the lines of expression, as I would were you in my consulting-room. Mine has reached your ears as a lone voice from the depths of some wilderness; I have tried so to speak with my pen that you could catch an echo as if from between the lines of every page.

You will not banish your medical adviser, for you still need his knowledge of the workings of disease, if you do not need the drugs you formerly believed necessary; but you will now be able in a more intelligent way to diminish the possibilities of the future need of him.

Since these wonderful fasts in Philadelphia others are occurring over the country from the contagion of example. Many are certain to be undertaken as a last resort where hope has departed; and death will come; and then there will be the confusion of tongues, as in the case of Mrs. Meyer. Her case has been the third one that I know of where the press has spread the news of death from starvation.

I have given you the case of Mrs. Meyer that you may know that no matter how hopeless any case may be considered, no matter how given up by venders of drugs, if a fast be advised and death come, death from starvation will be the general verdict. Hence on as fasts multiply, so will the press continue to make special note of all who chance to die because they had ceased to add distress to their bodies by foods that were only taken as the medicinal dose. All this you need to take into account in those cases you would advise where the medical faculty has retired in defeat.

Never in my entire professional life have I been so depressed by discordant voices as during this sixty-day fast just ended. All the air has been charged, darkened with frownings—even threats of what would happen in case of death; and as never before has this question come to me, "Why do the heathen rage and the people imagine vain things?"

Again I must tell you that the No-breakfast Plan, the plan not to eat in time of health until there are a normal need and desire for food, that are only developed after several hours of morning labor, and not to eat at all during acute sickness, is the easiest of all means to maintain health, and to regain it when lost. In my message I have had the greatest good for the greatest number of the world's busy people, who have no time to indulge abnormal, artificial ways in the recovery and maintenance of health—ways that are a real tax on time and taxing in the means involved. Passing few are they of the world's workers who have the time for all this, and especially they who are the slaves of the kitchen.

Again I must suggest to you that the actual need of daily food as a matter to meet the actual daily need is a new question in practical physiology. It may be very much less than is supposed, a matter to be determined by the scales. There are none who can eat at all with relish who are not more governed by relish than the hunger sense, as to the amount of food eaten. The real amount of daily food needed may be so small that enough of nourishment can be extracted from almost any of the easiest available foods, the main question being one of slow eating, restful eating, and with the most thorough mastication. For those who have the leisure and tastes for study over what to eat there are the works of Haig, Hoy, Hensel, Sir Henry Thompson, and others, that may be read with both interest and profit.

And now I address my last words to the mothers of the land. For you the No-breakfast Plan means the highest possible health, the greatest possible relief from the slavery of toil. On no other plan are there such promises of relief and prevention of all your sex ailings. On this plan only can you become man's equal in the hours of leisure that are his by a feeling of divine right; you also should consider the possibilities of a day of eight or ten hours as needing the reduction all the more because of your weaker bodies.

The No-breakfast Plan means for your children the best possibilities for the conservation of all the higher instincts and powers that will tend to save them from the saloon, the prison, the electric chair. If the Garden of Eden was abolished because you enticed man to eat the wrong food, it is for you to restore a new race of Adams in all the ways of health, of such health as will make the entire earth a "Paradise regained."

Readers, lay and professional, let me reiterate in my parting words, words at white heat with conviction as to their soundness and utility. Enforced food is a danger always to be measured by the gravity of the local or general disease; a danger always to be measured also by the feebleness of old age—by feebleness no matter how caused.

This physiological righteousness will remain unquestioned, its practicality unsurpassed, while man remains on the earth to violate the laws of his Creator manifest in his own body. The penalties of disobedience are as certain as that every cause is followed by a definite effect. There are no remissions in the various antitoxins; there is no hope for you through hollow needles. Nature is exacting, but she is merciful. Obey her laws that your ways may be toward Paradise, and not away from it.

www.ingramcontent.com/pod-product-compliance
Lightning Source LLC
Chambersburg PA
CBHW080022110526
44587CB00021BA/3739